Handbook to Health

Includes Menus and Easy to Prepare, Healthy, Tasty Recipes Everyone Will Enjoy Whether You are an Omnivore or Vegetarian.

Vivian Rice and
Edie Wogaman

Revised and Edited by
Julia L Wright

Photographs by:
Julia L Wright
Bob Wogaman

To request permission for reproduction:
email: info@handbooktohealth.com

This book is dedicated to
all of our clients,
who have also been
our teachers.

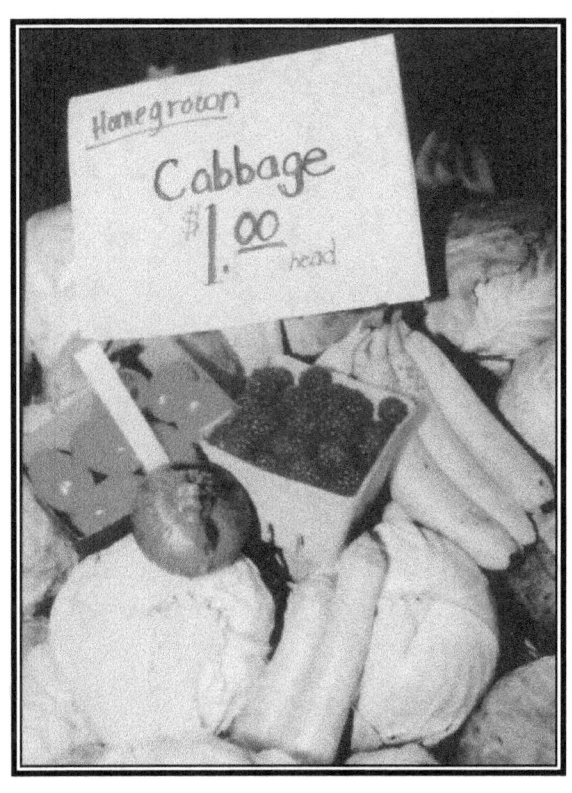

Acknowledgments

We have many people to thank for their patience, support, guidance and help in completing this and the original book.

Judy Ekstrom shared her cabin in the woods so that we could spend quiet, uninterrupted hours writing.

Marion Mabe spent endless hours at the computer typing and retyping our many changes.

Vivian M. LeFebvre was our proofreader, organizer and critic. She was our constant reminder that people reading this book have not had 35 and 20 years of experience, respectively, of living this lifestyle. She also designed the cover and interior, and prepared the final layout for the original publication.

We are grateful to our readers, **Colette and J.P. Monat**, for assisting with corrections before publishing.

Julia Wright for editing and creating this revised edition of Handbook to Health to share to a broader spectrum of people looking to change their life and create optimum health.

We thank **Burgess Market** in Tahlequah, OK, for allowing Bob Wogaman, of Heirloom Photography, to take the cabbage photograph.

Last, but not least, we thank our clients for their encouragement and insistence that we put this information into book form.

Within this book,
we provide nutrition education and
encourage self-help to prevent problems.

We do not practice medicine
nor diagnose or treat any disease.

May your life be blessed
with WELLNESS
by reading
and following
the suggestions in this book.

Introduction

This book is the result of requests by many clients, and years of questions from those clients, about how to start and end their days with the most nutritious and tasty foods.

The purpose is to inform you that there is an easy way to change your thinking and increase your health.

As always, we encourage each individual to be tested by a health professional who uses kinesiology (muscle-testing) to determine the most perfect diet that suits your body.

It is our intent to introduce you to a lifestyle change that you can easily accomplish. Throughout the book we recommend that you use the highest quality foods possible or available. Organic produce, drug-free and hormone-free animals and their by-products (such as organic butter), and farm-raised fish and shrimp are ideal.

If it is not possible for you to buy organic produce or to raise it yourself, the alternatives are to purchase your produce at a local farmer's market or use specific cleaning techniques to remove pesticides and herbicides. *(see Vegetable And Fruit Washes, pg. 22)*

We provide menus and correlating recipes to clarify and simplify what has become a very confusing approach to wellness. We offer appealing, tasty recipes with easy-to-find ingredients, that are time efficient for a busy schedule.

TO CONTACT VIVIAN
1900 East Pikes Peak Ave. Suite #8
Colorado Springs, CO 80909
Phone (719) 635-5596 • Fax (719) 635-5597
e-mail: wildrice3@juno.com
For supplements and herbs call
Nutraself—(719) 633-3056

VIVIAN RICE

NUTRITIONIST

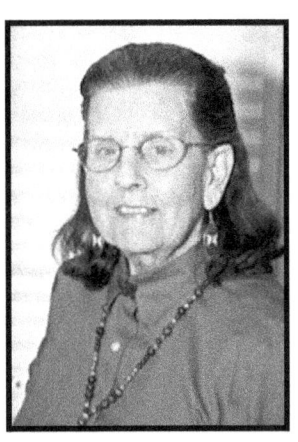

Vivian Rice began her professional career in 1964 as an LPN. Her experience working in hospitals as well as her personal experience with allergies motivated her to study and implement holistic healing methods.

She studied at the American Hygienic Society in Chicago, IL and at Dr. Shelton's Health School in Texas with a focus on nutrition. She also has studied with Paavo Airola, ND, in Arizona and with N. W. Walker Ph.D, in California.

She became a Certified Hypnotherapist and later graduated as a massage therapist and foot reflexologist.

Vivian became a Certified Healing Dialogue Therapist in 1983, and has done extended independent studies in nutrition, herbology and applied kinesiology. She has had more than 45 years experience in natural healing with nutrition and herbs. In 1980, Vivian opened and continues to operate her own healing practice.

A nationally known ceremonialist, educator and speaker, she is an active member of the American Holistic Nurses Association, The American Herb Guild, and the Pikes Peak Herb Association.

Vivian lives what she teaches. In 1983, she honored her Seminole Indian blood by learning and living the Spirit Road that honors all of the Creator's life forms and their synergistic purpose. She was adopted by the Lakota White Hawk family, in South Dakota.

TO CONTACT EDIE
1933 Timberline
Colorado Springs, CO 80920
www.ColoradoSpringCoaching.com
Phone (719) 531-0511
e-mail: pnut1943@att.net

EDIE WOGAMAN
COUNSELOR

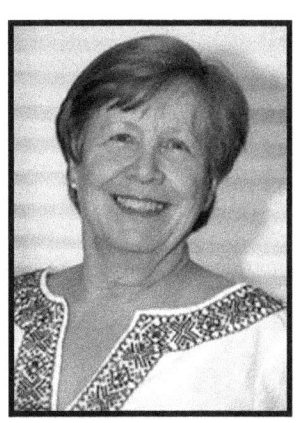

Edie Wogaman has been counseling in nutrition and lifestyle changes for thirty years. She has had intensive, supervised training in body chemistry balancing, personal growth, and communication issues.

In addition to her mental health counseling, Edie is a Certified Hypnotherapist, a Reiki II practitioner, and has completed all necessary training in EMDR (Eye Movement Desensitization and Reprocessing). Her Coaching training was with the Coaching Training Institute, California. This unique system assists one in having a happy, purposeful and successful life.

Her current training and certification is in Matrix Energetics, which is a form of quantum healing for every level of physical, emotional and spiritual concerns.

Edie's use of counseling skills, together with her vast knowledge in nutrition, creates a supportive blend that helps her facilitate clients' healing in body, mind and spirit.

Edie's practice keeps her traveling to the Southwest, as well as maintaining an established practice in Colorado Springs.

For more details on the counseling that Edie offers and schedule a consultation, visit her web site at:

www.ColoradoSpringsCoaching.com

Disclaimers

The information in this book is not intended to diagnose, treat, cure, or prevent any disease.

This manual is not intended to provide medical advice or to take the place of medical advice and treatment from your personal physician. Readers are advised to consult their own doctors or other qualified health professionals regarding the treatment of medical conditions.

The authors shall not be held liable or responsible for any misunderstanding or misuse of the information contained in this manual or for any loss, damage, or injury caused or alleged to be caused directly or indirectly by any treatment, action, or application of any food or food source discussed in this manual.

The statements in this book have not been evaluated by the U.S. Food and Drug Administration.

To inquire about private nutritional consulting or speaking engagements, contact:

Vivian Rice
1900 East Pikes Peak Ave.
Colorado Springs, CO 80909
Phone (719) 635-5596 • Fax (719) 635-5597
e-mail: wildrice3@juno.com

Edie Wogaman
1933 Timberline
Colorado Springs, CO 80920
www.ColoradoSpringCoaching.com
Phone (719) 531-0511
e-mail: pnut1943@gmail.com

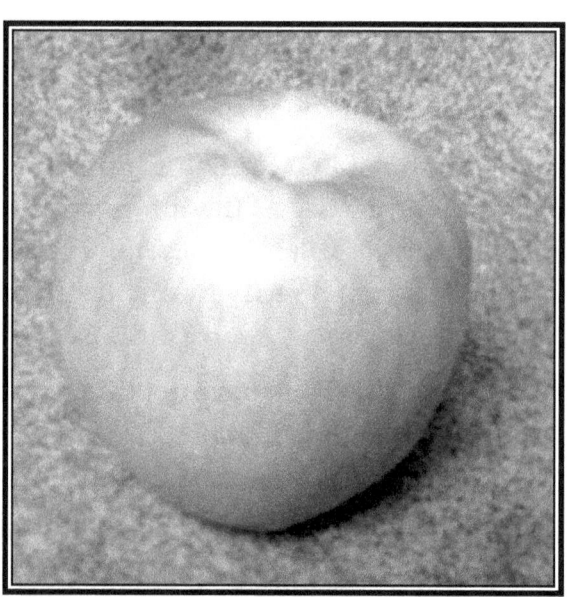

Contents

Chapter 5
Recipes 69

Appendix 137

Recipe Index 147

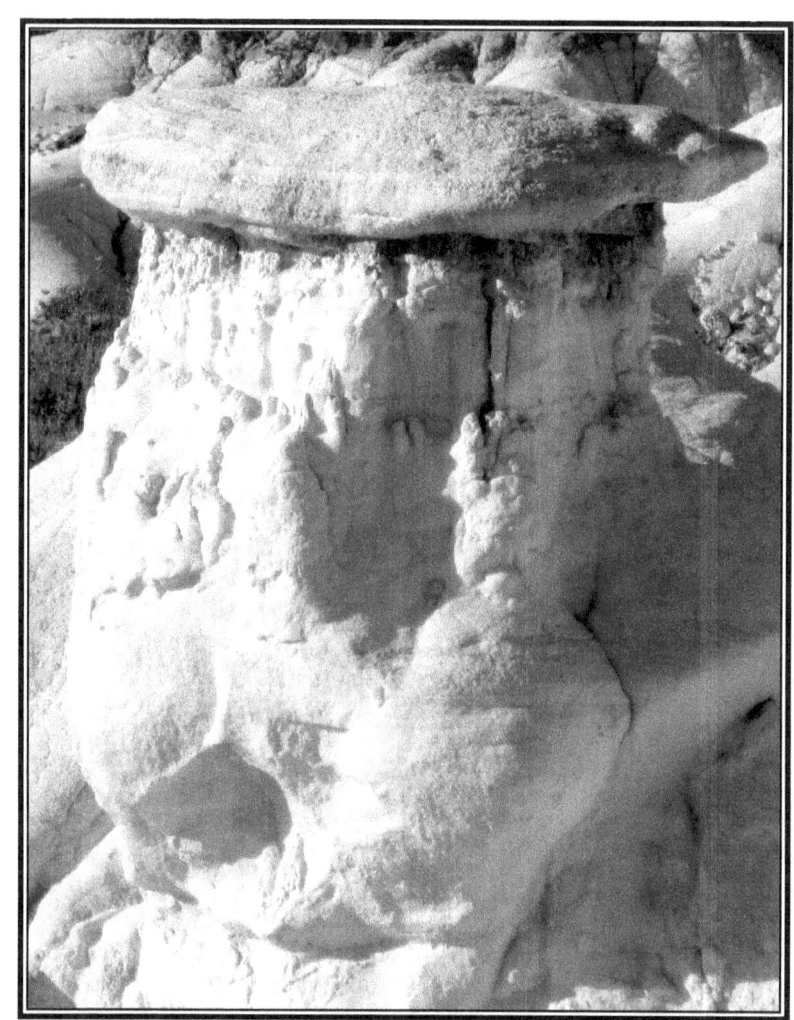

Chapter 1

Principles of Healthier Living

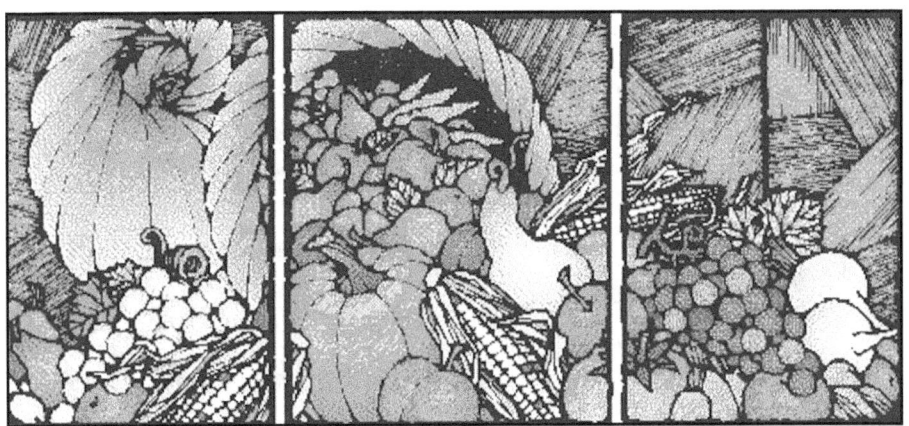

SOME BASICS

You are embarking on a course of "open mouth, insert nourishment."

The guidelines and menu ideas in this book will help you get the most out of the food you eat.

Eat foods in their natural state instead of refined. Ideal foods are organically grown.

Tap water in most cities has too much chlorine (which can contribute to thyroid dysfunction), sodium (which may elevate blood pressure) and aluminum (which may contribute to Alzheimer's Disease). Use distilled, natural spring or purified water.

Bottled water labeled "purified" or "drinking" could be tap water. Read the label for information on how the water has been purified. Osmosis (charcoal purification) is acceptable. Purified water in your home is important, especially if you have a water softener since many water softeners use salt.

Daily intake of viscous (slippery) herbs and foods nourish the colon and intestines, making the job of nutrient assimilation more efficient. These include slippery elm, coltsfoot, mullein, comfrey leaf, chia seeds, flax seeds and okra.

Small, frequent meals require less energy for digestion, leaving more energy for assimilation, elimination and healing. Small, frequent meals can increase metabolism.

All of the Recipes found in this guide have been tested by us, and many friends.

The Recipes are all Delicious, Easy to Prepare and Very Healthy.

Each person is different.

Keep this simple.

REMEMBER: ORGANIC FOODS ARE ALWAYS YOUR BEST CHOICE!

If you can't find organic, use whole foods that are found in their natural state.

- Whole foods are found in nature and have not been altered or added to by man or created in a factory.
- Free-ranging, grass fed animals or ones fed using an organic grain diet are healthier than commercially raised animals.
- Fresh food is better than frozen.
- Frozen is better than canned.
- If you buy canned foods, always check out the ingredients first.
- Chose Non-GMO foods.

When reading labels, remember these rules:

- Look at the Ingredients *before* you look at Nutrition Facts.
- If a food has an ingredient you cannot pronounce - Don't eat it!
- If it was not here hundreds of years ago - Don't eat it!

Enzymes

What Are They?

Enzymes are protein molecules that need helpers to fulfill their functions. One group of enzymes needs trace minerals. Another group needs organic compounds called co-enzymes. When a co-enzyme is tightly attached to the protein part of the enzyme, it is called a prosthetic group. Neither the co-enzyme nor the protein part of this prosthetic group can function alone. Co-enzymes consist of vitamins, especially the B vitamins. If you do not eat enough B-vitamin foods, these prosthetic groups cannot function efficiently. Disease is the result. This co-enzyme function applies to the enzymes that need trace minerals in your diet.

Enzymes are easily destroyed by heat (above 120°), acids and alkalines, as are many vitamins, especially water-soluble ones. This is why raw vegetables are better than cooked, soft ones. The live enzymes in raw foods help with digestion of the particular food.

Where Are Digestive Enzymes Found in the Body?

In the mouth amylase breaks down starches and sugars.

In the stomach the enzymes pepsin and HCL (hydrochloric acid) break down meat and/or vegetable protein into amino acids.

In the small intestines the metabolization process continues with the digestion of amino acids. Lipase breaks down the fats. Most enzymes are released by the pancreas. Bile from the liver digests salts and fats.

Enzymes at Work in Other Cultures

Dr. Edward Howell maintains that many people in Third World countries have great energy reserves because of eating traditional autolyzed, or predigested foods, developed long ago by their ancestors. The partially digested — i.e., fermented — food gives eaters more endurance, he says.[1] The reason for the effectiveness of autolyzed food, which has already been broken down into peptones and proteose, is it requires less of our personal digestive enzymes. Proteose is the intermediate product of proteolysis between protein and peptone.

Traditional foods predigested by enzyme processes include *kebbeh* from Lebanon, which is mostly raw lamb and crushed wheat. Wheat and lamb are pounded together for about an hour, kneaded, seasoned and eaten raw.

Dr. Howell says that the enzymes cathepsin-D and lipase in the lamb, along with protease, amylase and lipase in the wheat, are liberated during the pulverization process. The enzymes then work together to achieve predigestion and deactivate the enzyme inhibitors during the time of pulverization. "Therefore," he says, "the predigestion continues both before and after food is eaten, until the stomach acidity becomes very strong."

Certain fungal enzymes are used by Asiatic people to promote predigestion of proteins, carbohydrates and fats during the food preparation process. Other foods include tofu, a vegetable cheese made from soybeans with the help of fungal enzymes; miso, a Japanese specialty improved by enzymatic action on soybeans, rice, or barley; and tempeh, a soybean enzyme food from Indonesia. Examples include the Chinese dishes *tofu kan, tofu p'i* and *yuba*.

---

[1] *Dr. Edward Howell, Enzyme Nutrition, Wayne Avery Publishing Group, Inc., 1985.*

Food Combining Chart

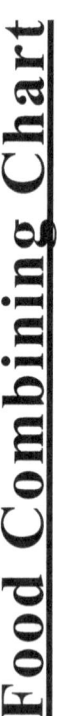

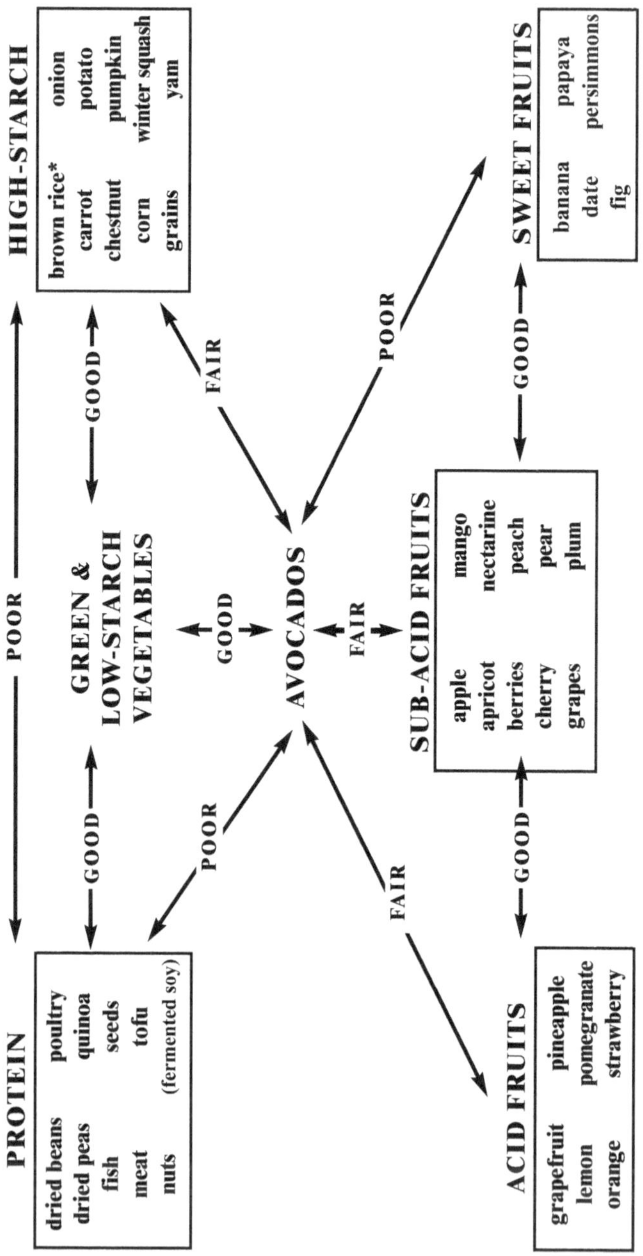

HIGH-STARCH

brown rice*	onion
carrot	potato
chestnut	pumpkin
corn	winter squash
grains	yam

GREEN & LOW-STARCH VEGETABLES

PROTEIN

dried beans	poultry
dried peas	quinoa
fish	seeds
meat	tofu
nuts	(fermented soy)

AVOCADOS

SUB-ACID FRUITS

apple	mango
apricot	nectarine
berries	peach
cherry	pear
grapes	plum

SWEET FRUITS

banana	papaya
date	persimmons
fig	

ACID FRUITS

grapefruit	pineapple
lemon	pomegranate
orange	strawberry

PROTEIN — HIGH-STARCH: POOR
PROTEIN — GREEN & LOW-STARCH VEGETABLES: GOOD
GREEN & LOW-STARCH VEGETABLES — HIGH-STARCH: GOOD
HIGH-STARCH — AVOCADOS: FAIR
HIGH-STARCH — SWEET FRUITS: POOR
GREEN & LOW-STARCH VEGETABLES — AVOCADOS: GOOD
PROTEIN — AVOCADOS: POOR
AVOCADOS — SUB-ACID FRUITS: FAIR
AVOCADOS — ACID FRUITS: FAIR
SUB-ACID FRUITS — SWEET FRUITS: GOOD
ACID FRUITS — SUB-ACID FRUITS: GOOD

Food Combinations

Proper food combining is the key to changing body chemistry to maintain good health and proper body weight. See the Food Combining Chart located to the left and on page 142 in the Appendix.

- Eat fruits *only* with other fruits.

  (See the Food Combining Chart to the left.)

- Meats, fish, fowl, well-cooked grains or starchy vegetables, such as squash, potatoes and corn, are best eaten with raw or steamed green vegetables.

---

*Brown rice is an exception to the poor High-Starch/Protein relationship; it digests well with animal and vegetable proteins.

Eat only one concentrated protein food at a meal.

Tomatoes may be combined with low-starch vegetables and nuts or avocados.

Fruits should be eaten as a fruit meal, unmixed with other foods except lettuce and/or celery.

Melons should always be eaten alone.

Dangers of Dairy

Milk contains the enzyme phosphatase which is necessary to metabolize calcium. Pasteurization kills this and all other enzymes in the milk. This is one of the reasons why calcium in pasteurized cow's milk is not properly utilized by humans.

Cow's milk is altered for human consumption; i.e., the protein content is diluted with water, and the carbohydrate content is increased with dextrose or corn syrup (instead of milk sugar). Acid (special culture) is added to make a finer curd in cottage cheese. Consequently, cow's milk products cause an alkaline reaction in the colon instead of an acid reaction as human milk would, which may lead to congestion of dairy products in the colon, and cause an allergic reaction.

Elevated serum uric acid levels in adults can be traced to cow's milk and cheese.

Some processed cheese made in the United States has too little natural bacteria to aid in its digestion. Chemicals are used to speed aging. European cheese and/or naturally aged cheese retains the needed digestive bacteria and is, therefore, healthier to eat. These cheeses are aged to grow healthy bacteria (similar to acidophilus in yogurt, which aids in assimilation). Yellow dye #5 put into some "yellow" and "orange" cheese removes Vitamin B6 from the body, which can cause finger joint pain. The loss of B6 also reduces serotonin levels in the brain. Many orange cheeses (Colby, cheddar, etc.) use "annatto" for coloring. Annatto is an acceptable vegetable coloring.

The calcium and protein in cows' milk is intended to build the bones and bulk of a 1,200-2,000-pound animal. Human milk has less protein and more carbohydrates by volume than animal milk. This fact indicates that humans need less protein than animals, except for pregnant mothers and athletes. Medical researchers are realizing the human protein requirements are much less than the beef and dairy industries promote through the U.S. Federal Drug Administration (FDA). For more information on this topic, read *Food for Fitness*, written by George Beinhorn, published by Anderson World, and the article "Milk!" in *Discovery* Magazine, August 2000.

Raw goat's milk is closer to human milk chemically and, therefore, more easily digested by infants. Goats do not get the diseases cows do, consequently, they do not need the same vaccinations as cows. Nanny goats are clean, especially with regard to what they eat; the same cannot be said of Billy goats.

Mothers:
Please Nurse Your Babies!!!

The enzymes in your milk are essential for your children's physical, mental and emotional health.

Your body also needs that hormonal stimulation from your pituitary gland to complete the birth and lactating cycle. Nursing causes contraction of the uterus restoring its muscular integrity.

If for some reason you cannot nurse, raw goat's milk from a reliable source is second best and closest to your human milk and nutrients.

GOAT MILK SOURCE:
Ask your local health food store for sources.

Low-Stress Foods

Always try for organic produce

- Vegetables, preferably raw
- Steamed foods are always considered to be less stressful to the body, due to the enzymes needed for digestion, still being available.
- Raw seeds and nuts
- Fish
- Vegetable juices
- Organic fruits
- Avocado
- Sprouted grains
- Beans
- Organic condiments, such as mustard, cider vinegar, horseradish
- Poultry (skin removed), especially drug-free
- Brown rice

Fatty Acids
Essential for complete amino acid assimilation

It is best not to eat margarine due to trans-fatty acids, which are hard on the liver—especially canola margarine.

Canola was one of the first genetically engineered plants. There is no such thing as organic Canola oil and it is no longer considered an acceptable oil to use for cooking. It is actually considered to be toxic. *(Source: Dr. Mercola)*

Trans-fatty acids are created by overheating fats and are to be avoided

In preparing the oil mix or butter-oil mix, be sure to use the oil and amount that agrees with your current food sensitivity.

Oil Mix

Mix three tablespoons of wheat germ oil or flax seed oil into three cups of cold-pressed oil, such as safflower, extra virgin olive, sunflower or soy (soy has more Vitamin E). Refrigerate after opening as all oils become rancid rapidly, except extra virgin olive oil.

Butter-Oil Mix

Mix one pound of organic, sweet cream, unsalted, pasteurized butter with 1-1/2 cups of oil.
Sea salt may be added if you do not have a salt restriction.
Blend and refrigerate.

*In warm climates, use 1/4-1/2 cup less oil.

The best oils to use are organic, cold-pressed oils.

Cold-pressed oils are made by first grinding nuts, seeds, fruits or vegetables (depending on the oil being made) into a paste. Then an oil stone or other tool is used to press the paste which forces the oil to separate out.

Expeller-pressed means it is heated. Heat damages oils.

Recommended "Good" oils to use when cooking are Organic, Cold-Pressed: Extra Virgin Olive *(dark green color)*, Safflower, Sunflower, Sesame or Coconut oil.

Coconut oil has Loric Acid, so it is comparable to human mother's milk. Loric Acid is microbial. It also contains cholesterol fat which is why It is solid at room temperature. It should be kept in the dark, but not refrigerated.

You can find all of these at your local Health Food store.

Eat And Enjoy

- Well-cooked (low heat) whole grains that have been soaked, as well as sprouted grains.

- Raw, fresh fruit. Peel apples and pears if not organically grown. Pesticides are in the skin and will not wash off.

- Raw nuts and seeds. Chew all nuts until they are liquid. When you buy nuts and seeds, taste one to ensure freshness.
  If you prefer roasted nuts and seeds, do it yourself. *(pg. 70)*

- Raw or organic sweet cream, unsalted, pasteurized butter.

- Occasionally, white or annatto-colored cheese, aged 100 days.

- Steamed, baked, grilled or broiled chicken, turkey, fish or seafood, preferably organic beef, pork, lamb and buffalo. Deer and elk may be eaten.

- Raw vegetables assist the digestion of cooked food because they provide live enzymes.

- Raw, steamed, baked, grilled, broiled or sautéed vegetables.

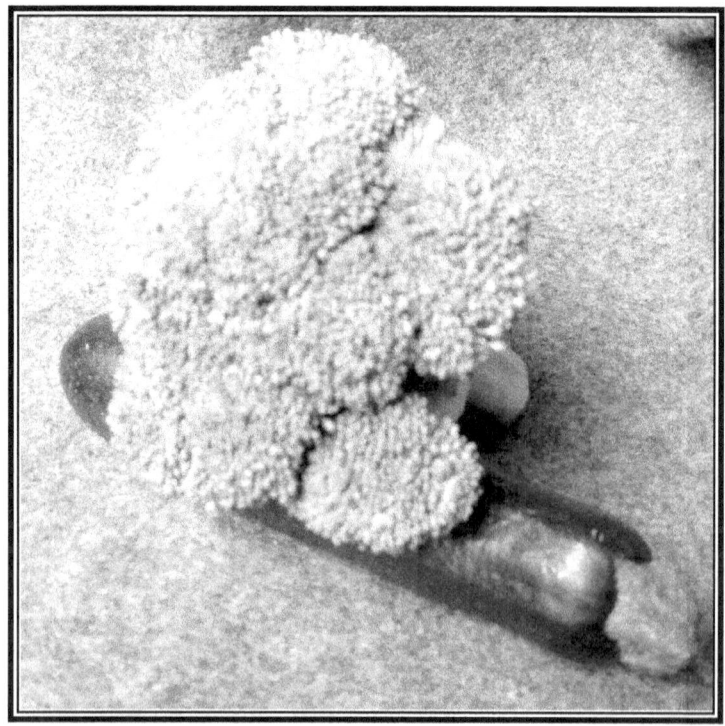

- Bottled or frozen fruit juices (except citrus) without added sweeteners. Dilute juices at least one-half with purified water.

- For a treat, try frozen rice drink ice cream, soy ice cream, tofu puddings or gelatin dessert (vegetable gelatin).

- Experiment with tempeh, soy milk, soy cheese, tofu, and rice or almond cheese.

- Drink green tea and decaffeinated herbal teas.

- Sprouted flourless bread, which digests like a vegetable.

- Starchy vegetables with meats, fish, fowl or well-cooked grains overtax the digestive system. An exception is brown rice which may be eaten with animal protein.

- Dairy products are best eaten with raw or steamed green vegetables, never with fruit, honey or other sweeteners. *Except for stevia* (sweet herb), never combine dairy products with fruit, honey or sweeteners because a protein vs. sugar digestion battle rages in the stomach.

- Mixing a dairy product, sweetener or fruit with oatmeal results in a chemical change that can cause putrefaction in the blood, skin problems, and excess gas.

- Oatmeal can be eaten with sweet cream, unsalted butter; salt; spices, such as anise, cardamom, cinnamon or coriander; herbs, such as fennel, sweet basil or stevia; and/or pure vanilla flavoring.

- Whole grains are best eaten the same way as oatmeal or with vegetables (sautéed, stir-fried or in soups and stews).

- Melons, be sure to eat separate from other foods and fruits to reap the most benefit.

High-Stress Foods

High-stress foods require greater digestive energy,
and can also cause allergic reactions

- Beef, pork and their by-products
- Coffee, black tea and caffeinated soda
- Condiments (pickles, catsup, soy products such as high sodium soy sauces, mayonnaise, syrups, etc.)
- Refined sugar and refined flours and grains
- White potatoes
- Tomatoes
- Brewer's Yeast
- Dairy and ice cream products
- Alcohol
- Margarine
- Syrups with artificial color and flavor
- Sweetened fruits and juices with artificial color and flavor
- Hardened shortenings
- Packaged, commercial gravies
- Most nuts, especially dry-roasted, salted nuts
- Organ meats, especially liver
- Chocolate
- White distilled vinegar
- Artificial colors, flavors, monosodium glutamate and preservatives.
- Overcooked vegetables. Overcooking converts the starch to indigestible carbohydrates, destroys water-soluble vitamins and oxidizes fat-soluble vitamins, thereby placing this form of vegetable into the High-stress Food category.

Avoid

- Fried foods should always be avoided. Highly heated fats create trans-fatty acids, which are indigestible.
- Any and everything that contains aspartame sugar substitute. These substances become methyl alcohol at 88°F. Your body temperature is approximately 98.6°F.
- Irradiated foods and microwave ovens. It is better to use a convection oven.
- Eating any refined and processed foods, especially anything made white by processing, such as sugar, flour or vinegar.
  If it's white, take flight! This includes white bagels, muffins and pastries.
- Artificial colors, flavors, monosodium glutamate and preservatives.
- Combining or following any meal with fruit or sweets. Sugar interferes with the complete breakdown of proteins and usually leads to gas.
- Fish with broccoli. This combination does not digest well. The cause is unknown.
- Eating commercially raised cow and cow products, lamb or veal. Also, avoid commercial salted or unsalted butter.
- Eating pork, ham, bacon or any part of a pig, due primarily to fat, salt and chemical content.
- Drinking caffeine products, such as coffee (regular or decaf), soft drinks, black tea, chai tea or chocolate. Caffeine overstimulates all body functions and can increase fibroids. Soft drinks also have high phosphorus content, which contributes to osteoporosis.
- Iceberg lettuce (also called head lettuce).
- Drinking bottled, canned or frozen citrus juices. The rind carries an oil-based insecticide spray that can be toxic to the liver. Make your own citrus juice, without squeezing the skin unless organically grown.
- Drinking liquids with meals, because it inhibits maximum digestion. Four to six ounces of water for taking supplements is allowable. Otherwise, water consumption should take place 15 minutes before and 30 minutes after meals.
- Genetically engineered/modified (GMO) foods. These are not labeled, which is another good reason to eat whole, organic foods. Some "organic" packaged foods use irradiated spices and herbs because the FDA does not require labeling on combination foods, only whole foods.

Why Not Caffeine?

Caffeine in coffee, black tea, caffeinated sodas and chocolate on a daily basis interferes with the central nervous system and hormonal function.

Caffeine overstimulates the central nervous system, which causes an instant overstimulation in the pancreas, raising the insulin level to excess, which lowers blood sugar rapidly. This helps create hypoglycemia, which is a factor in Attention Deficit Disorder (ADD), mood swings, hot flashes and night sweats for men and women.

The same overstimulation causes the adrenal glands to secrete too much aldosterone, which can raise the sodium level, causing water retention.

The antioxidant properties in green tea seem to negate overstimulation by its caffeine component.

Dietary Change Cautions

You may or may not experience changes, such as withdrawal or detoxification (the removal of toxins or poisonous effects from your body), during the first few days or weeks of your nutritional program.

- Reducing coffee gradually will prevent withdrawal headaches.
- Not eating wheat can cause drowsiness or a feeling of being tired if you are wheat-sensitive.
- Diet changes and/or supplement intake can increase the number of stools and/or lead to loose stools.
- Detoxification may cause a temporary increase of gas.

Note: As a result of extreme cross breeding of wheat and genetic changes, wheat is no longer the nutritious grain that it was originally.

Emotions And Spirit

Most of this book focuses on physical nutrition, with menus and recipes to assist you in creating the best possible health you can experience. It is important, also, to focus on the other aspects which are a part of the entire picture called you. We have mentioned the vital part that exercise plays in your well-being. Take a close look at what makes up your emotional outlook and what spiritual connections you have.

Take time each day to check your current outlook on life. Have an awareness of the status of your relationships. Are they satisfactory or do they need improvement? Educate yourself. There are many useful tools and systems that you can find in self-help books or in conversations with professionals.

Lift your spirits with the things in your life that make you smile. Help yourself feel more connected to your individual spiritual beliefs. Use practices you are most comfortable with, or create new ones that fill your heart and soul.

Physical Activity

Muscles are made for motion, therefore, movement is their greatest need. Lack of physical activity can atrophy the muscles, as well as the mind and the emotions.

Exercise is a VITAL part of our health (whether we like it or not). It is "quality of life" that is referred to here. Exercise can take many forms. We tend to think about exercise in terms of calisthenics, running, working out at a gym, or squeezing it into our busy day. We often dread making a daily commitment to our bodies.

Exercise can be meditative. It works toward toning at the same time. Swimming, hiking, bicycling and walking are great methods of exercise. Tai chi, yoga, and Qi Gong are other possibilities. Dancing is a wonderful, playful type of exercise that works the body and has great cardiovascular and emotional benefits. Remember the most recent time you danced and how good it felt.

Get the blood circulating and the heart pumping. Deep breathing tones the internal organs and stimulates the adrenals. Our digestive and elimination systems also work more effectively when we exercise regularly. When we move our bodies our thirst increases and we drink more water, which gets another part of our elimination system going.

Whatever form of physical activity you choose,
get started today**!**

Questions And Answers

Q: How do I get started, and what about all the food in my pantry?
A: Simple! Slowly and gradually incorporate whole foods into each meal.

Q: Isn't organic food more expensive?
A: Not in the long run, especially if you eat out a lot. Organic will actually be less expensive compared to the cost of medicine such as aspirins, tranquilizers, antacids, allergy medications, and lactose intolerance aids.

Q: Doesn't shopping for and cooking whole foods take a lot of time?
A: Healthful eating requires a change in your priorities. Just remember, you are worth it.

Q: Are there special foods I should eat each week?
A: Whole foods should be eaten every day.

Q: Can I ever go out to dinner?
A: It is more expensive, both financially and bodily, to eat out. However, more and more restaurants are becoming health-conscious. Some use organic foods and some are gluten-free.

Q: Can I shop and cook ahead to make life a little easier?
A: Of course. You can cook ahead whether from scratch or a package-type meal. Check out the convenience food section in the health food store.

Q: Is breakfast really that important?
A: Yes, it is! Breakfast begins the metabolism in the body.

Q: Can I ever have any desserts and sweets?
A: Yes, you can. There are several suggestions in this book.

Q: Sometimes after lunch I am too sleepy to work. Can you tell me what is happening?
A: This is usually caused by too many carbohydrates for breakfast and lunch.

Q: How do I keep motivated to maintain a healthier diet?
A: By the high levels of energy, positive outlook, and more youthful appearance obtained from eating whole foods.

Q: What do food cravings mean?
A: Craving sugar, caffeine and refined foods indicate negative addictions. We also crave things because it is something our body wants or needs at a certain time. This is a positive, nonaddictive craving we need to heed.

Q: What is tofu? Tempeh? Why are they so good for me?
A: These are fermented soy products. If you test well for soy, its isoflavones support the heart and circulation. The phytoestrogens can assist hormone balance.

Q: Is fasting recommended?
A: Only with guidance from your health care provider.

Q: I like to snack. What's good for me?
A: There are many snacks suggested throughout this book. *Check out the a snack section on pages 37-39.*

Q: Can eating healthily help me lose weight?
A: It can help keep your weight in balance.

Q: How can I overcome constipation?
A: Pinpoint and eliminate the foods that block, such as refined flour and sugar. Increase intake of water and foods high in magnesium and potassium. *For suggestions, refer to the Vitamin Charts (pp. 140-141) and Mineral Chart (pg. 143) located in the Appendix.*

Q: Can changing what I eat help me with insomnia?
A: Yes! Several things can cause insomnia, including alcohol, caffeine and late-night eating. Hormonal imbalance may also be a factor.

Q: How can I get more energy?
A: Changing your diet to live foods will immediately increase your energy level.

Q: Will healthy eating help me live longer?
A: Keeping physically active, eating live, whole foods, and maintaining a positive attitude can make a difference.

Chapter 2

FOOD PREP, ZEST AND PLANNING

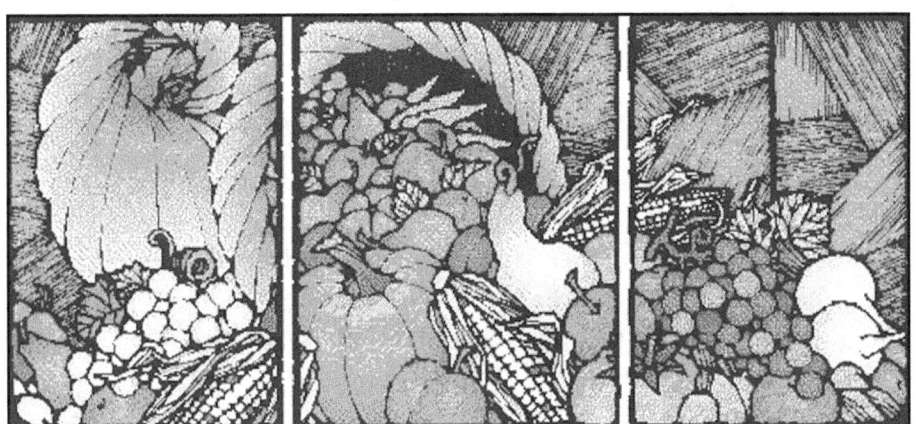

Convenience Cooking

One of the most important things to remember is to prepare double or triple amounts of food, which makes your life much easier later.

Divide food into meal-size portions to provide you with healthy options on those days when you come home feeling tired, or your day has just been filled with busyness.

Cooking for more than one meal enables you to have prepared meals that you can freeze for future use. There are only a few foods that do not freeze well such as those with high-water content as cucumbers, tomatoes, and pears.

With a little extra forethought, it is possible to provide healthy meals for you and your family with very little extra effort.

Using weekend days for planning menus, shopping and food preparation, makes the entire week more pleasant.

With only a small amount of time and effort you can plan meals that not only meet nutritional guidelines, but are tasty as well.

Prepare two chickens instead of one, doubling the amount of rice and steaming several different vegetables.

Select your meal for that evening. Use the remaining food for future meals. *For example,* soups or stews, or freeze for another day.

When cooking ground turkey, make two meat loaves or several batches of meatballs. This way there is plenty left for lunches or a variety of meals for the coming week.

Extra rice can be used for a stir-fried breakfast the next morning, or added to a batch of vegetable soup. Freeze food in individual servings.

When cutting fruit for a snack or meal, clean and cut extra and freeze some for a smoothie drink or Fruit Crisp Dessert. *(page 130)*

Encourage your children to get involved with food planning and preparation. This gives them an opportunity to be involved in their own well-being, as well as providing great parent-child togetherness time.

Valuable learning can be shared and experienced, not only about foods and good nutrition, but about your child's thoughts and feelings.

Vegetable And Fruit Washes

- 2 tablespoons sea salt in 1 gallon of cold water

- Bleach Wash:
  1 capful bleach to a sink full of cold water
  Soak 5 minutes
  Rinse in clear, cold water

- Organic produce only needs to be rinsed in plain water.

Herbs And Spices

Spices and herbs make food more nourishing while changing the flavor of "the same old vegetables."

Let your nose teach you how to flavor your food. Smell the food and then the herb. When the aromas blend, it tastes good as well.

Salt *(preferably sun-dried, noniodized sea salt)* and pepper *(black, red or white)* are best added at the table.

High-heat cooking causes a molecular change that makes pepper indigestible and hard on the kidneys. Uncooked black pepper has a glucose tolerance factor that helps digest sugar.

Suggested Flavoring Spices

allspice	ginger
anise seed	Italian blend
bay leaf	lemon balm
black pepper (uncooked, freshly ground)	marjoram
caraway	mint
cardamom	nutmeg
cayenne	oregano
cinnamon	paprika
chervil	rosemary
cloves	saffron
cumin	sage
cilantro	salad herbs
coriander	summer savory
curry	sweet basil
dill	thyme
fennel seed	sorrel

or any spice your Grandmother would use

Chapter 3

CHANGING COURSES

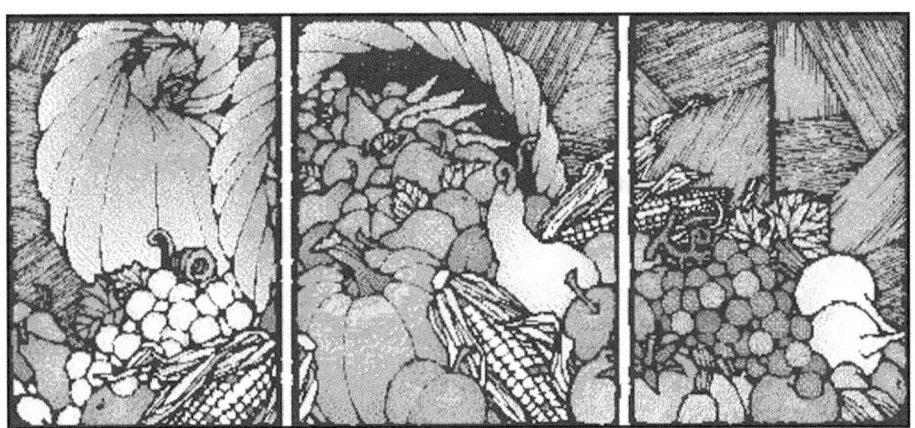

Breakfast

Your first meal of the day breaks the fast of sleep time. The nutrients you give your body at breakfast begin the process of metabolism, which provides energy throughout the day.

Live foods, such as salads, raw vegetables with eggs or other cooked proteins, give your body live enzymes to assist in better digestion.

Eggs and animal proteins have no fiber; vegetables, grains and fruit have fiber. It is commonly known that fiber is vitally important in keeping the digestive system healthy and cleared of waste. In the menus you will see the proper way to combine foods.

The menus in this book will help you change your belief system that there are only certain food combinations eaten for breakfast, lunch and dinner.

The concept of American breakfast foods comes from the media. The strong advertising is from companies who produce dairy products, frozen and boxed sweets, and is directed toward our children. This makes it difficult for parents to help children make healthy choices.

It is important to have our cupboards and refrigerators filled with nutritious foods from which our children can choose.

Please remember there are plenty of other foods to eat in the morning besides those we consider breakfast foods. Leftovers from dinner the night before is a favorite of ours; especially stir-fried vegetables and brown rice or soups or stews.

Cooked whole grains that your body can tolerate are yummy breakfast options. Eat them with a salad or some raw vegetables and you will feel satisfied and nourished.

There are many vegetarian "meat" flavors and substitutes made from grains, and many soy products that can fill in the blanks when you desire variety.

It is hard for some people to consider, but think about it. If you perceive that nourishing your body in the morning is the goal, what you choose really makes a difference.

You can be certain that all processed cereals, donuts or fast-food breakfast items will take away from your body rather than replenish it after the night's rest.

People who work night shifts have learned to eat any meal at any time. **It is important to avoid solid food between midnight and 4 a.m.** During these hours the pancreas releases specific protein enzymes to eliminate floating cancer cells. If food is consumed during this time, these protein enzymes will have to digest food instead of cancer cells.

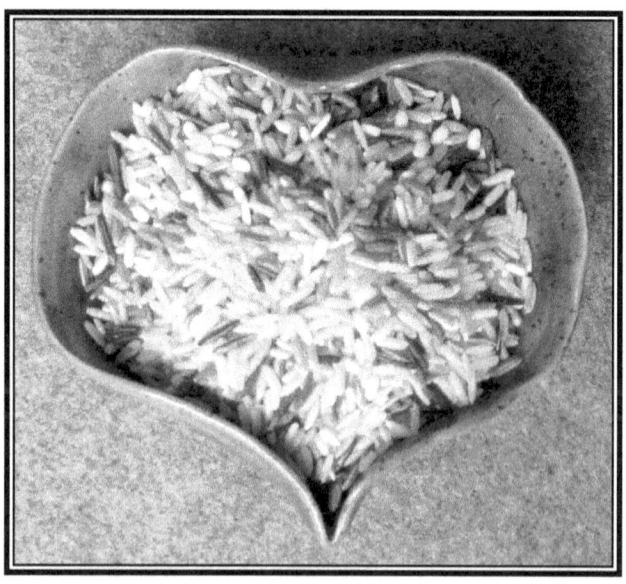

Breakfast Possibilities
Add raw green vegetables to protein and grain meals

- Poached eggs with raw celery or spring salad and toasted sprouted flourless bread.
- Eggs steamed in nest of precooked brown rice.
- Serving of well-cooked whole grain (millet, oat groats, cream of rye, barley, cream of buckwheat or brown rice), cooked on medium/low heat, which leaves more nutrients intact. It is not necessary to presoak cream of buckwheat, cream of rye, bear mush, or steel cut or rolled oats. Do not use milk or sweetener, especially with oatmeal. Use soy milk, almond milk, rice drink or oat milk. Use butter-oil mix (pg. 11) and sea salt. It is best to eat green vegetables with this.
- Turkey breakfast sausages and eggs with sprouted flourless toast or spelt toast and 1 or 2 romaine leaves.
- Scrambled eggs with turkey bacon and sprouted flourless bread or spelt toast, and celery sticks or salad.
- French toast made with sprouted flourless bread or spelt bread, topped with sweet cream butter, sugar snaps or peas.
- One or two soft-cooked eggs with green salad or celery sticks, sprouts or any raw vegetable of your choice and sprouted flourless toast of your choice.

- Egg omelet with any of these sautéed vegetables:

bell pepper	bok choy
spring salad	cucumber slices
dandelion leaves	young Swiss chard
onion	zucchini
sugar snap peas	romaine leaves
red Russian kale	sweet basil (herb)
broccoli	raw or cold green beans
celery	small amount of kelp
garlic	raw or cold snow peas

  red cherry tomatoes are also acceptable

Season at the table with sea salt and pepper.
Enjoy with sprouted flourless or oat bran toast.

- One-half to one ripe mashed avocado, plain or with lemon and sea salt, salsa or organic mustard, on sprouted flourless toast.
- Eggs and brown rice.
- Tossed green salad (no head lettuce) with dressing of oil mix (pg. 11) and lemon or vinegar (cider, rice or balsamic), or plain yogurt and one of the following:
  Sprouted flourless bread
  Spelt bread
  1-3 unsalted rice cakes or wafers
  3 slices flat bread
  1 slice of bran bread
  1-3 white corn or whole grain sprouted flourless tortillas
- White, aged cheese and salad with raw wheat germ. Only eat sprouted flourless bread or rice crackers with cheese.
- Homemade granola without fruit.
- Fruit plate. Remember citrus with citrus, melons with melons. *(See Food Combining Chart, page 142.)*
- Under certain, rare conditions in a restaurant, dry cereal with no sweeteners added, is acceptable using cream, half and half, or good water.

Before Breakfast Possibilities
(per your health practitioner recommendations)

- Take any special teas or supplements
- Juice of half a fresh lemon or lime plus a scant amount of cayenne pepper in a full glass of warm water for ongoing cleansing of the body
- Grapefruit
- Fruit in season
- Decaffeinated herb teas such as Country Apple, Chamomile, Lemongrass, Mandarin Orange, Sleepytime®, Ginseng Plus or drinks as Pero, Cafex or Roma, Teeccino
- Black cherry juice or cranberry juice diluted by one-half with water for kidney support

Beverages used for cereals, baking, cooking or drinking are: Rice Dream, Amasake, soy milk, oat milk and almond milk. *These beverages are not for infants or babies up to two years of age.*

Early Riser/Light Eater
(Those inclined to skip breakfast)
Remember to add some greens

- Nut butter on sprouted flourless toast
(hazelnut, almond *or organic peanut butter, if no peanut allergy)*
- Handful of nuts or seeds
- Small bowl of grains, e.g., oats, brown rice, barley, quinoa
- Hard-boiled eggs
- Sprouted flourless toast with mashed avocado and choice of sliced tomatoes or lemon juice or mustard
- Protein Drink *(pg. 40)*

Lunch

At Home

Planning meals saves time, money and your health. You can prepare soups, stews and casseroles in advance in weekly quantities and freeze them. Freeze in serving sizes. Thaw overnight for sandwiches or burritos for lunches for the next day.

Weekends are a good time to cook soups and stews in a crock pot. This gives you time to cool, separate and freeze them the next day.

Electric steamers are also indispensable in our kitchens; be certain the parts that touch the food are plastic. Avoid aluminum cookware.

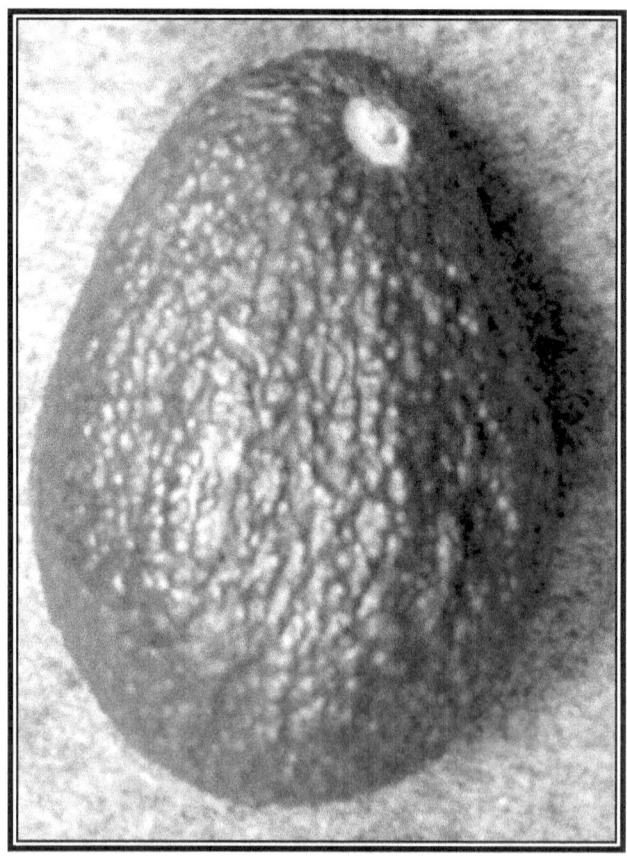

More About Lunch

- 1-2 cups of sautéed vegetables—choose from:

  | bell pepper | cabbage | celery | garlic | onions |
  | parsley | radishes | sweet potato | | |

Cook with anise seed or sweet basil. After cooking, season with seasoned salt, sea salt, tamari, or tofu sauce. Pour over 1/2 to 2 cups of well-cooked brown rice.

- Sautée 1-2 cups of vegetables listed above. Instead of using brown rice, add salsa and roll into tortillas.

- 1/2 to 2 cups of boiled barley, brown rice or millet, topped with a sautéed choice of:

  | bell pepper | bok choy | celery | garlic | kale |
  | onions | zucchini or yellow crookneck squash | | | |

Season with sweet basil or coriander. Serve with a small green salad with oil mix (pg. 11) dressing.

- Baked or steamed squash, such as:

  | banana | hubbard | spaghetti |
  | zucchini | yellow crookneck | |

- Top spaghetti squash with Italian tomato sauce or natural pasta sauce. *Serve with whole grain sprouted flourless bread, celery sticks, a whole baked onion, and a green salad with oil mix* (pg. 11) *dressing.*

- Steamed vegetables. In steamer, layer some quartered potatoes with parsley, carrots (sliced lengthwise and sprinkled abundantly with sweet basil), cabbage in eighths or quarters sprinkled with rosemary or marjoram, then onions *(herbs are optional)*. Steam 15-20 minutes, turn off heat, do not lift lid and let stand 10 minutes. Pour on some butter-oil mix (pg. 11). *Serve with sprouted flourless bread and a tossed salad.*

- Baked, grilled, steamed or broiled fish seasoned with garlic, parsley, whole allspice berries, sweet cream unsalted butter and lemon or lime. *Serve with a small green salad and/or baked vegetable and fluffy brown rice.*

- Baked, skinless turkey or chicken, stuffed with whole onion and zucchini, celery and garlic. *Serve with some steamed green vegetables, fluffy brown rice, a small salad, and sprouted flourless bread.*

Six-day Lunch Ideas

MONDAY

Soy Pizza Slice
1 slice sprouted flourless or whole grain toasted bread
Pasta sauce (pg. 122 for sauce without tomatoes)
1 slice soy cheese
Suggested toppings:
   olives, mushrooms, zucchini, roasted red bell peppers,
   pepperoni, artichoke hearts.

Cover toast with pasta sauce.
Add cheese and 2-3 of your favorite toppings.
Apply pasta sauce to toppings.

Bake in toaster oven at 350° for 5-10 minutes, or until cheese melts.

Warm up lunch even more with some Pearl Barley Vegetable Soup (pg. 80)
and green tea.

TUESDAY

Chicken Sandwich
2 slices sprouted flourless bread
Slices of drug-free chicken
Mayonnaise

Nibble along with romaine leaves dipped in your favorite salad dressing;
sip some herb tea.

WEDNESDAY

Avocado Vegetable Sandwich
2 slices whole grain bread or sprouted flourless bread
Eggless mayonnaise or stone ground mustard
1/4 medium-large avocado, sliced
Cucumber, seeded and thinly sliced
Lettuce, romaine or leaf

Enjoy with leftover cold yam or sweet potato.

THURSDAY

Peanut Butter* Cucumber Sandwich
2 slices sprouted flourless bread
Organic Valencia peanut butter*
Cucumber or celery, thinly sliced and peeled

Enjoy with mixed baby greens salad with homemade dressing, and/or celery sticks.

*Note: If allergic to peanuts, substitute almond or hazelnut.

FRIDAY

Grilled Cheese Sandwich
2 slices whole grain bread or sprouted flourless bread
Butter-oil mix (pg. 11)
American-style soy or rice cheese

Butter the sides of the bread that will touch the skillet.
Grill over medium-low heat until golden brown.

Enjoy with a tossed salad and hot or cold Teeccino (caffeine-free herbal coffee).

SATURDAY

Taco Lunch
1 large romaine leaf wrapped around the following:
1/4 mashed avocado
1/4 cup sunflower seed sprouts
Dash with a small amount of picante sauce or lemon juice, and cumin.

Brown Bag Lunches

Sprouted flourless bread is best because you can use any filling; meats digest well with sprouted flourless bread.

Remember, leftovers make great lunches!

More Sandwich Ideas

- Vegetable pocket from the health food store
- Turkey
- Egg Salad *(pg. 82; pg. 91 for Tofu Egg-free Egg Salad)* with thinly sliced onion and lettuce
- Tuna salad made with white albacore tuna
- Avocado with sprouts and tomato
- Nut butter (almond, cashew, Valencia peanuts)
- Almond, soy or rice cheese

Sandwich Sides

- Raw vegetables
- Baked chips (sweet potato, carrot, potato— *no corn*)
- Fruit
- Potato salad
- Cole slaw
- Soup
- Raw nuts
- Organic pretzels

Dinner

- Grilled chicken, turkey or fish
  Steamed vegetables, such as green beans, onions and zucchini
  brown, forbidden, black, red or wild rice
  Salad
- Chicken Stew *(pg. 106)*
  Mixed green salad
- Chicken and brown, forbidden, or basmati brown rice
  Spelt bread
- Chicken Paprika *(pg. 104)* with brown, forbidden, or basmati
  brown rice
  Steamed asparagus
  Mixed salad greens
- Easy Curried Chicken *(pg. 104)* with steamed rice
  Steamed fresh green beans
- Grilled Dilled Salmon *(pg. 113)*
  Steamed spinach
  Mixed salad (try spring salad for a change—little preparation
  and big taste)
- Grilled Chicken Salad with Thai Noodles *(pg. 82)*
  — Thai noodles are made from rice
- Turkey Meat Loaf *(pg. 108)*
  Asparagus and onions
  Cabbage salad or coleslaw
- Ground Turkey Meatballs with Gravy *(pg. 110)*
  Spelt pasta
  Choice of steamed broccoli, Swiss chard or mixed salad
- Steamed vegetables, such as carrots, potatoes, beets, onions,
  celery, green beans, cabbage
  Mixed green salad
  Texas-style sprouted flourless toast
- Tossed green salad with sprouts, jicama, raw zucchini, and other
  salad ingredients—except no iceberg lettuce, and top with oil
  mix (pg. 11) and lemon dressing
  Choice of sprouted flourless bread, spelt bread or 1-3 rice cakes

- Homemade Vegetable Soup *(pg. 79)*
  Sprouted flourless bread
- Raw vegetable sandwich using sprouted flourless bread (or sourdough), add sprouts, mushrooms, cucumbers, tomatoes, leaf lettuce, imitation mayonnaise
- Grace's Turkey Soup *(pg. 75)* or chicken soup with brown rice Garnish soup with 1/2 cup of steamed, sliced sprouts before serving
  Whole rye bread
  Green vegetables
- Cabbage, carrot, beets and onion with dill weed, rosemary, lemon and oil
  Choice of sprouted flourless bread, spelt bread, 2 rice cakes, flat bread, bran bread, tortillas, or homemade bread

----

Snacks
Midday, Midafternoon and Early Evening

Protein Snacks

- Celery sticks with nut butter (cashew or almond)
- Turkey or chicken wrapped in lettuce leaves
- Leftover chicken or turkey pieces eaten with greens
- Bowl of leftover beans and brown rice
- Raw almonds, walnuts or seeds
- Soy milk

Carbohydrate Snacks

- Cold sweet potato or yam
- White or blue popcorn
- Brown rice cakes
- Whole grain crackers, seeded or nut crackers
- Raw or cooked fruits
- Raw carrot sticks, broccoli, cucumber, celery, snow peas, red potatoes, turnips, cabbage, daikon or other radishes
- Wheat-free waffles with fruit-sweetened jam or jelly
- Rice drink ice cream bars or sandwiches
- Carob-covered raisins
- Artichoke leaves dipped in your favorite healthy dressing
- Dry cereal (oats without sugar) eaten dry

Mid-morning Snacks
Two hours after breakfast

- 6 ounces of carrot juice mixed with 2 ounces of any green vegetable juice and
4 ounces of water.
- 3 ounces of carrot juice mixed with 3 ounces of water.
- 1-3 celery sticks stuffed with any nut butter
(roasted or raw; salted or unsalted):
choose almond, cashew, sesame, *or Spanish or Valencia peanuts, unless allergic to peanuts.*
- 1-2 tablespoons of presoaked (for easier digestion) seeds. Soak in just enough water to be absorbed with very little, if any, water left.
- Sunflower seed butter with raw green vegetables.
- Organic fresh fruit in season—must be ripe.
- Any raw vegetable (except cauliflower, which may interfere with thyroid function).
- 1-3 cups white or blue popcorn, lightly salted with noniodized, sun-dried sea salt or nutritional yeast.
- Organic dried fruit reconstituted with water.
- Bowl of any cooked grain (millet, oats, cream of rye, bear mush, barley, brown rice)
with cinnamon, ginger, nutmeg or coriander to flavor the grains, along with celery sticks or any raw vegetable
- Leaf artichoke dipped in oil mix (pg. 11), or lemon and herb, such as chervil or dill
- Baked potato with oil mix (pg. 11) or butter-oil mix and sprouts—mushrooms *(optional)*
- Sprouted flourless bread sandwich with safflower mayonnaise— use turkey, chicken, eggs or tuna and greens
- Green salad with nondairy dressing

Mid-afternoon Snacks
At least two hours before dinner

- Fruit plate
- Baked, unsalted chips
- Raw nuts
- Raw vegetables

One Hour Before Bed

- 1 cup sprouts
- 1/2 avocado
- To prevent low blood sugar in the morning, have 1/4 or 1/2 cup of any cooked grain—except wheat—or a slice of sprouted flourless toast
- Goat yogurt with bran or sprouts
- Fresh fruit, unless hypoglycemic

Beverages

- Green tea (Caffeine in green tea is milder. Green tea has antioxidants and less caffeine.)
- Grain drinks
- Soy milk
- Rice drink beverages
- Oat milk (Oat drink is not recommended due to sugar content.)
- Almond milk
- Raw goat's milk
- Organic fruit or vegetables juices—dilute by one-half with purified water
- Herbal teas
- Purified or distilled water

Protein Drink

1 rounded tablespoon rice protein drink powder
  or 1 rounded tablespoon non-GMO soy protein powder
1 tablespoon raw almonds or 1 tablespoon raw pecans
2 tablespoons sesame seeds
1 tablespoon chia seeds
8-10 ounces rice drink, soy milk, almond milk or water

    Pour 1/3 cup of liquid in a blender.
    Add powder, nuts and seeds.
    Process until well-blended.
    Add remaining liquid and blend again.

Sweets

*The best time to eat sweets is
at least two hours before or after a meal*

Sweets can fit into your life as a treat or a meal.
For example, use a fruit plate as a meal or as a snack between meals. The very best sweets are the live, nutritious ones known as raw fruits. Some people require cooked fruits.

If cooked or raw fruits cause gas, essential enzymes required to break down sugars and fibers are missing from the body's digestive process to break down the sugars and the fibers. Digestive enzymes may be taken to assist digestion.

Most familiar dessert recipes are not properly food-combined. There are methods to rearrange familiar recipes, with the substitutes listed in this book, which are far more digestible. For instance, use oat milk, soy milk or almond milk instead of dairy.

The best flours are organically grown whole wheat pastry flour, spelt flour, barley flour, potato flour and tapioca flour.

Sugars that can substitute for refined white sugar are succanat, local honey, pure maple syrup, blackstrap molasses, cane juice or syrup, brown rice syrup and barley malt.

White fructose usually comes from corn rather than fruit. *Many people are corn-sensitive.*

Sweet Ideas

- Blended frozen fruits make great sorbets. Adding rice beverages makes it a creamy dessert.
- Health food stores carry great gelatin desserts.
- Substitute fruit cobblers for pie. Fruits can also be used for puddings.
- Fruit pie sweetened with fruit juice.

Whole organic grains make tasty desserts. Use them when making cookies, sweet breads, bread pudding, rice pudding or cakes.

See Sweets And Sweet Ideas recipes *(pp. 128-135)* for more healthy ways to soothe that sweet tooth.

NOTE: **If you begin your day with something sweet, all day long you will eat, and eat and eat.**

Chapter 4
Specific Menu Plans

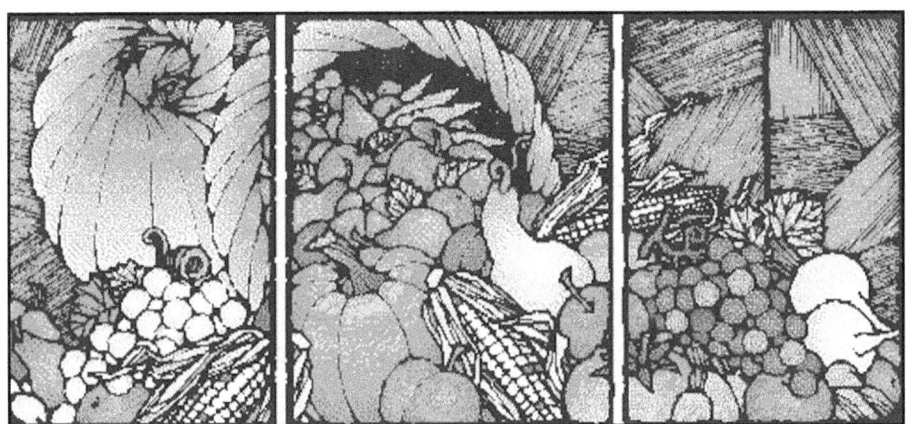

Candida

Candida Albicans is a naturally occurring yeast or fungus that belongs in our bodies.

Candida increases when we get out of balance by not dealing properly with the stress in our lives, and/or intake of daily doses of refined foods, alcohol, caffeine, chocolate, sodas, and taking birth control pills or antibiotics.

The Candida increases itself in mucous layers in the small intestines. These layers prevent any nutrients from nutritious foods from getting into the bloodstream, which normally carries nutrients into the muscles.

Ninety percent of the metabolism of nutrients is meant to occur in the muscles.

This is why Candida in excess is a major contributing factor to chronic fatigue syndrome, fibromyalgia and Epstein-Barr virus.

Foods that feed this condition are dairy (except butter), flour (especially wheat), corn, refined sugar, chocolate, coffee, peanuts, alcohol and beef—not necessarily in that order.

The most difficult meal for those with excessive candida is usually breakfast.

Most traditional breakfast foods are high in carbohydrates.

Follow the suggestions in these Candida Breakfast Menu Plans.

Candida Breakfast Menu Plans

No fruit before 2 p.m.

• **Egg omelet with vegetables sautéed in a good cold-pressed oil** (pg. 11) **or water.**
Choose 3 from:

broccoli	garlic	peas
bok choy	green beans	celery
green cabbage	mung sprouts	parsley
Napa cabbage	onions (green)	radishes
zucchini	green or red peppers	
tomatoes (cherry or Roma are best)		

Sprouted flourless toast with small amount of unsalted, sweet cream butter.

• **Eggs fixed your favorite way**
Sprouted flourless toast
Something raw and green

• **Cold chicken**
Sprouted flourless toast
Celery sticks

- **Long or short grain brown rice.**
  Cook in double boiler: 1 part rice to 2 parts water.
  Have one of the following with cooked rice:
  Soy milk with cinnamon and sea salt
  Small amount of butter, sea salt, dill weed and sweet basil
  Small amount of butter, sea salt, poached or scrambled eggs
  Seasoning of your choice, celery sticks and/or lettuce leaves
  Salad with lemon and oil

- **Tofu scramble for those with egg sensitivities.**
  Take tofu from water pack and allow to dry overnight on a rack,
  towel or paper towel. If cut into large slices, it dries faster.
  Sauté small amount of garlic or onion and parsley.
  Add crumbled tofu and scramble.
  Sprouted flourless toast.

- **Cream of buckwheat.**
  With a small amount of sweet cream butter and sea salt
  Add soy or almond milk

- **For the long-time vegetarian:**
  Tossed salad with chia, sesame or sunflower seeds, or any nuts
  except peanuts
  Sprouted flourless toast with small amount of butter-oil mix (pg.
  11)

- Protein Drink *(pg. 40)*

Chronic Fatigue

Chronic Fatigue Syndrome refers to fatigue that develops slowly and persists for a long period of time.

Causes of the fatigue are exhaustion or loss of strength from excess physical activity; an emotional state linked to extreme or extended exposure to psychic pressure, as in battle or combat.

"Any bite of food
that is not health-giving
is health-destroying."

The Uncook Book, page 31

Hypoglycemia

Hypoglycemia is also known as low blood sugar.

The symptoms are low energy, poor memory and concentration, confusion, anxiety and mood swings.

Adherence to our hypoglycemia food plan has helped many people eliminate hypoglycemia.

There are a few important concepts to remember.

To avoid putting sugars into an already sugar-sensitive body, morning foods must be protein or complex carbohydrates; e.g., whole grains, such as brown, forbidden, or basmati brown rice.

Carbohydrates and sugars should only be ingested during midday (2:00-4:00 p.m.), and only once per day. The body metabolizes carbohydrates and sugars best at that time of day.

Hypoglycemia is caused by too much insulin in the bloodstream.

Research has proven that caffeine in coffee, black tea and chocolate elevate the insulin level. This is why eliminating caffeine altogether is essential in bringing balance to the pancreas, where insulin is made.

Starting the day with a protein drink, such as, brown rice powder or soy powder, or a protein breakfast, slowly releases insulin.

Balancing the protein with green vegetables normalizes the blood sugar.

Whole grain crackers and breads are complex carbohydrates that release sugars into the bloodstream slowly. Refined grains become instant sugar, which rapidly raises the insulin level.

Specific Menu Plans

Hypoglycemia And Chronic Fatigue Menu Plans

DAY 1

Breakfast
Turkey sausages and eggs
Sprouted flourless toast
1-2 romaine lettuce leaves

Mid-morning
Celery with nut butter (almond, hazelnut)

Lunch
Grilled chicken salad with dressing of extra virgin olive oil and fresh lemon juice
Sprouted flourless bread or brown rice

Mid-afternoon
Raw or cooked fruit

Dinner
Grilled Dilled Salmon *(pg. 113)* or baked salmon
Steamed asparagus
Salad or brown rice

DAY 2

Breakfast
Vegetable omelet using 1-3 eggs
Sprouted flourless bread
Raw green vegetables

Mid-morning
Sprouted flourless bread with nut butter (almond, hazelnut, or organic peanut butter, if no allergy to peanuts)

Lunch
Chicken, Brown Rice and Green Bean Soup *(pg. 76)*

Mid-afternoon
Raw nuts or seeds

Dinner
Stir-fried vegetables with choice of: shrimp; drug- and hormone-free beef, buffalo or chicken
Brown, forbidden black, or red rice
Salad, if you choose

DAY 3

Breakfast   French toast made with sprouted flourless bread
Butter and/or cinnamon
Green vegetable of your choice

Mid-morning   Bowl of cooked whole grain (brown rice, quinoa or amaranth) cereal or whole grain crackers

Lunch   Turkey burger on sprouted flourless bread
Mustard, sugar-free mayonnaise or unsweetened catsup
Salad

Mid-afternoon   Raw vegetable sticks or baked potato with butter

Dinner   Chicken Stew *(pg. 106)*
Brown, forbidden black, or basmati brown rice
Salad

NOTE: Fish may be used instead of chicken or turkey.

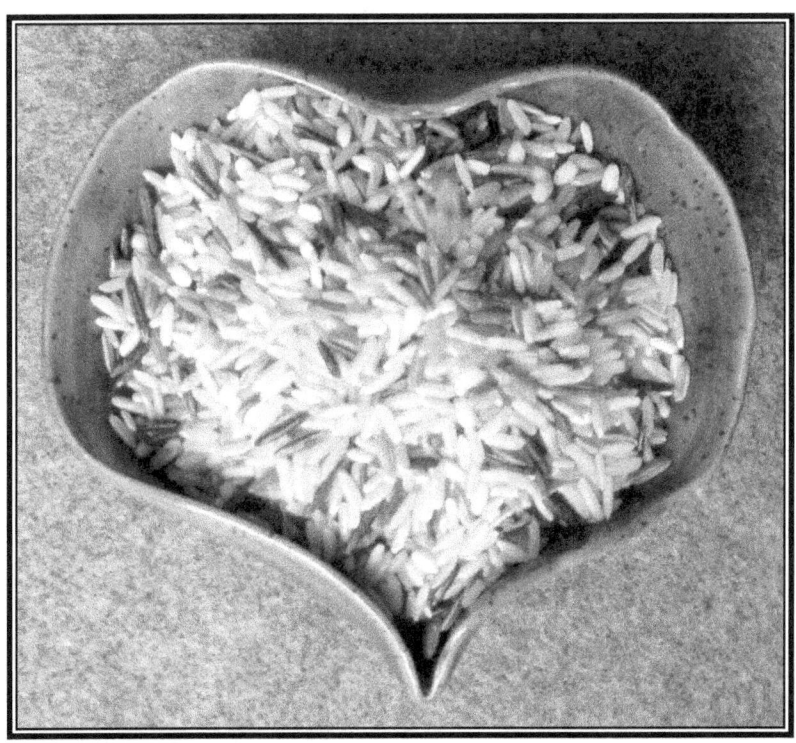

Hypoglycemic Vegetarian Menu Plan

Hypoglycemia elimination is managed with a high-protein diet, as well as focusing on assisting pancreatic function with proper food intake. Vegetarians usually need increased education in order to prepare high-protein meals.

Breakfast Precooked brown rice with black beans, seasoned with your favorite herb; e.g., sweet basil, dill weed, cumin or curry; extra virgin olive oil or butter-oil mix (pg. 11)
Slice of organic sprouted flourless bread with Gomasio *(pg. 69)*
Unsweetened soy milk, sweetened with a few drops of stevia

Mid-morning Slice of organic sprouted flourless bread with nut butter (almond or hazelnut)

Lunch Well-cooked whole grain couscous or quinoa
Salad with nuts or seeds, but no tomatoes
Toasted organic sprouted flourless bread

Dinner Sesame-Tofu Stir-fry *(pg. 125)*
Wild or forbidden black rice
Soy milk (unsweetened or sweetened with a few drops of stevia)

One Hour Before Bed
For Vegetarian and Non-vegetarian

Choose one:
- Slice of whole grain toast with thinly spread nut butter (almond or hazelnut)

- Whole grain cereal with or without soy milk

- Whole grain crackers with soy cheese

Suggested Herbs and Spices

allspice	ginger
anise seed	Italian blend
basil	lemon balm
bay leaf	marjoram
caraway	nutmeg
cardamom	oregano
cayenne	paprika
chervil	peppermint
cloves	rosemary
cumin	saffron
cilantro	sage
coriander	summer savory
curry	sweet basil
dill	thyme
fennel seed	sorrel

or any herb your Grandmother would use

High Blood Pressure

When the onset of high blood pressure has a simple physical cause, such as high caffeine and salt intake, then the food plans outlined can bring it down to normal.

If the physical cause is complicated, such as a brain tumor or kidney disease, then the following food plans are essential. When the body is compromised in this way, nourishment is essential to bring balance.

If high blood pressure stems from stress, then your daily intake needs to be large quantities of loving kindness to yourself first and everyone else next. Following a non-nerve-stimulating food plan helps take the stress off of your central nervous system and kidneys.

How does caffeine raise your blood pressure? It overstimulates your nervous system which in turn overstimulates your entire endocrine (glandular) system. Your adrenals then secrete too much aldosterone, which raises the sodium level in your blood. This, in turn, stresses your kidneys, which can raise your blood pressure.

Adding more salt to your food overloads the kidneys. The kidneys' main function is to filter toxins from the blood. When the blood carries excess sodium it can inflame the kidneys.

Purified water in your home is important, especially if you have a water softener since many water softeners use salt.

Avoid deep-fried foods, salt, caffeine and hot, spicy foods.

Use herbs for flavoring, such as dill, sweet basil, sesame seeds or celery seed.

High Blood Pressure Menu Plans

DAY 1

Breakfast

Poached or boiled eggs, seasoned with summer savory
Sprouted flourless toast with butter
Quinoa seasoned with oregano

Mid-morning

Unsalted almond or cashew butter in celery

Or

Mid-morning

Unsalted sprouted flourless bread sandwich with home-baked chicken
Mixed green salad

Mid-afternoon

Fruit of choice, e.g, organic apple or pear

Dinner

Grilled Dilled Salmon *(pg. 113)*
Brown, forbidden black, or basmati brown rice
Steamed asparagus
Sliced cucumbers

DAY 2

Breakfast

French toast (use sprouted flourless bread)
Romaine lettuce leaves with lemon and an organic, cold-pressed oil dressing
Green tea

Mid-morning

Raw almonds, cashews and/or pecans

Or

Mid-morning

Mixed green salad
Albacore tuna, water-packed
Rice crackers, salt-free

Mid-afternoon

Fruit of choice, e. g., organic apple or pear

Dinner

Vegetable Millet Soup *(pg. 81)*
Spelt Biscuits *(pg. 71)*

DAY 3

Breakfast   Steel-cut oats or cream of buckwheat
Sprouted flourless toast, buttered
Soy milk or rice drink
Green beans

Mid-morning   Sunflower seeds

Or

Mid-morning   Pasta vegetable salad on mixed greens
Unsalted sprouted flourless bread

Mid-afternoon   Leftover baked or grilled chicken

Dinner   Trout a la Vivian *(pg. 117)*
Wild rice
Steamed Swiss chard

NOTES:

• **Remember, to get live enzymes, always eat a raw green vegetable when eating protein.**

• **Remember most lunch meats and condiments are highly salted.**

Menopause

Menopause means the pause of menses.

It has come to mean much more to females.

Ideally, menopause is a time for us to lighten up on many habits that no longer serve us. Menopause is the shift from a time in our lives that was once filled with building careers and, for many, raising children.

Premenopausal years were a time of sending our energies out to the rest of the world.

Often the symptoms that women's bodies can experience are mood swings, hormonal swings, sporadic periods, heavy flow and insomnia. This distracts from what can be a time of introspection. Now it is time to change our lifestyle to avoid those negative experiences and to reinvent ourselves for the future decades.

Some foods can contribute to hot flashes and night sweats, and certainly to mood swings. These foods and beverages are dairy products (except for butter)—especially cheese of any kind—pastries, candy, chocolate, alcohol, beef, pork, lamb or buffalo, white bread and coffee. These are the very things women often crave. All interfere with a smoother ride through this time of your life.

Now that your children are older and in some cases, old enough to care for themselves, it can be easier to lighten your diet. Make healthier choices, put more fun into life, add efficient exercise (e.g., swimming, rebounding, brisk walking) and look at each day as a day that can benefit your health and well-being.

Lightening your diet means reducing the amount of flour, red meat, cheese and caffeine. Increasing live (raw) food intake is important. Eating smaller, more frequent meals, aids the body during hormonal shifts. Diminishing enzymes can be bolstered with plant enzyme supplementation, which can prevent dreaded weight gain.

Use some of the frustration that can come along with menopausal body changes to your benefit. Increase your repertoire of coping skills. Begin to shift your perspective of longstanding aggravations into new views that lift your spirits and make your life more joyful.

More frequent, lighter meals, properly combined foods and exercise allow you to gracefully cycle through menopause, rather than have menopause drive you off your life path.

Menopause Menu Plans
Follow the Hypoglycemia and Chronic Fatigue Menu Plans on pages 48-49.

Arthritis

Arthritis is swelling and inflammation of the joints.

There are two major types: osteo and rheumatoid.

Rheumatoid arthritis is an autoimmune disease.

Both involve the joints, cartilage, tissue and bone and are aggravated by an acid condition of the body.

Red meat (beef, pork, elk, deer, buffalo and lamb) is highly acidic and puts heavy stress on an arthritic body.

The energy output required to metabolize animal protein is extreme, which depletes the body's energy and ability to heal; therefore, animal flesh foods are best eaten at the noon meal.

The major portion of the food plan for arthritis is creating an alkaline/acid balance. Low-stress foods, especially organically grown, are alkaline-forming. *(See Low-stress Foods, pg. 10.)*

Nightshades, which are tomatoes, white (russet) potatoes, eggplant, bell peppers and spinach are exceptions to alkaline-forming vegetables. This is due to the nightshades' high oxacylic acid content.

The ideal is to be individually food-tested by a health practitioner, using kinesiology, because of the uniqueness of each body's chemistry.

It is important to shift your diet gradually.

Almost all traditional breakfast foods are acid-forming.

Open-mindedness to eating and trying new menu ideas will give the most relief from pain and swelling.

Important to note is that mental and emotional stress also contribute to an acid condition of the body. These mental and emotional stressors are anger, resentment, fear and impatience.

Arthritis Menu Plans

DAY 1

Breakfast Eggs
Sprouted flourless bread, buttered—no jelly
Raw green vegetable of your choice
Green tea or water (hot water with lemon is a good choice)

Mid-morning Raw nuts

Lunch Fish, steamed or baked
Steamed vegetables
Mixed green salad (with lemon juice and extra virgin olive oil dressing)

Mid-afternoon Apple or pear (peeled if not organic)

Dinner Stir-fried vegetables
Brown rice
Celery sticks or other raw vegetables

DAY 2

Breakfast Cream of rice with cinnamon and butter
Almond or soy milk
Sprouted flourless toast with butter-oil mix (pg. 11)

Mid-morning Rice crackers

Lunch Turkey sandwich on sprouted flourless bread with lettuce, sprouts and cucumbers

Mid-afternoon Peach or nectarine

Dinner Black beans and brown rice
Mixed green salad

DAY 3

Breakfast	Wheat-free waffles with butter
	Applesauce
	Green tea or hot lemon water
Mid-morning	Almond butter on celery or romaine lettuce leaf
Lunch	Chicken Stew *(pg. 106)*
	Rice crackers or sprouted flourless toast
Mid-afternoon	Plums
Dinner	Steamed vegetables (zucchini, sweet or red potato, green beans, onions)

NOTE: It is wise to eat flesh food only once per day, since arthritis thrives in an acidic body.

"Protein in sprouts has been converted to amino acids and as such is predigested."

The Uncook Book, page 50

Diabetes Type II

Type II diabetes is a mild condition, usually early or late onset, and usually can be healed through diet alteration.

It is possible to eat and drink your way out of diabetes, just like you ate and drank your way into it.

The major cause is unhealed mental and emotional stress.

Other causes for this condition include lack of physical activity; excess consumption of sugars, refined foods, artificial flavoring and coloring, fats, caffeine, chocolate and alcohol.

Learning methods to reduce stress is as important as the following food information.

One of the substances found in grains, particularly wheat and rye, is phytic acid. Phytic acid irritates the pancreas, which interferes with proper function. Therefore, we recommend the gradual elimination of wheat and rye from the diet.

The way to heal yourself of this condition is with dark green vegetables, such as kale, collard greens, spinach, mustard greens, chard, broccoli, beet greens and turnip greens.

Taking supplemental digestive enzymes with each meal is also essential.

Other foods that restore pancreatic function are blueberry leaf tea and raw (not dried) whole cranberries.

Stevia used as a sweetener helps regulate blood sugar. Add 2-3 drops of stevia to blueberry leaf tea.

Diabetes II Menu Plans

DAY 1

Breakfast
Brown rice
Eggs, poached or soft-boiled
Blueberry leaf tea

Mid-morning
4 raw cranberries (keep raw cranberries in freezer and thaw as needed)

Lunch
White albacore tuna salad
Mixed salad greens
Rice crackers

Mid-afternoon
Low-sugar fruit (tart apples or berries)

Dinner
Grilled or baked chicken breast
Steamed green Russian kale
Quinoa whole grain, seasoned with butter-oil mix (pg. 11) and herbs of your choice
Blueberry leaf tea

DAY 2

Breakfast
Turkey sausages
Sprouted flourless toast
Mixed spring salad
Blueberry leaf tea

Mid-morning
4 raw cranberries

Lunch
Baked yellow Yukon potato with butter-oil mix
Mixed green salad

Mid-afternoon
Organic fruit

Dinner
Striped Bass with Mushrooms on a Bed of Spinach (pg. 116)
Tomato and cucumber salad
Blueberry leaf tea

DAY 3

Breakfast   Chicken and Leek Soup *(pg. 75)*
                    Sprouted flourless toast, buttered
                    Blueberry leaf tea

Mid-morning   4 raw cranberries

Lunch   Steamed vegetables (Swiss chard, broccoli, turnip
                    greens)

Mid-afternoon   Raw nuts

Dinner   Ground Turkey Meatballs with Gravy *(pg. 110)*
                        Served on brown basmati rice
                    Steamed asparagus
                    Mixed green salad
                    Blueberry leaf tea

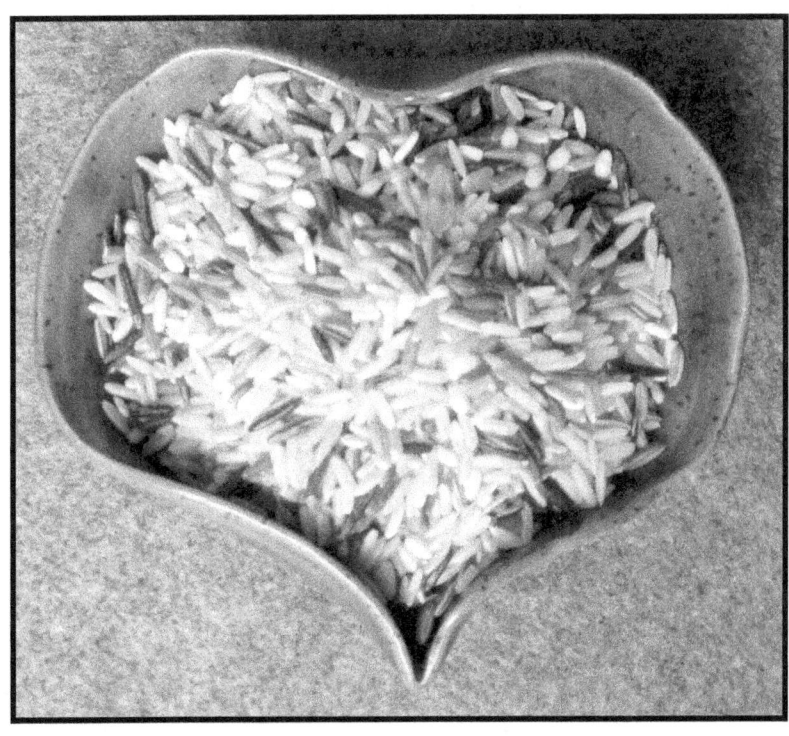

The Soy Controversy

The controversy over the safety of soy products has surfaced in recent years, and we want to address this from our experience. We have carefully observed, using muscle testing as well as tracking clients' results, how differently people respond to the various uses of soy in the diet, nutritionally and medicinally.

It is critical that the soy that you use is organic non-GMO (Genetically Modified Organisms).

More people can eat organic fermented soy products than soy products that are unfermented.

The Pros and Cons of soy, in our opinion, are:

Pros

The isoflavones in soy, primarily genistein and daidzein, have antioxidant and phytoestrogen properties. Our muscle testing has shown the mild estrogen activity of soy isoflavones can reduce and/or eliminate menopause symptoms without creating estrogen-related problems. The exception to this is if the person has a thyroid problem. She usually tests negatively on soy.

Iso (equal) flavones (ketone derivataries) and phytosterols in soy have anti-inflammatory properties. These are provided in concentrate in capsule form.

Soy can be a good protein source for adults, eaten in small amounts, one time per day. We emphasize this because traditionally those cultures of people who have lived successfully with soy in their diets for many generations eat their soy along with meat or fish, but rarely as the main source of protein in the diet.

Soy has an anti-protein digesting enzyme (trypsin inhibitor) which negates soy as a complete protein food. Vegetarians and vegans need ground, raw flax seeds or chia seeds to get all the eight essential amino acids required for new cell building. They can also eat whole grains, such as rice with beans to form a nearly complete protein.

Cooking destroys the amino acid lysine.

```
Soy Addendum
Reminder:
Always Use ONLY
Organic, Non-GMO Soy.
```

Cons

Soy can be difficult for some people to digest, resulting in gas and/or water retention.

Biochemist, Mike Fitzpatrick, PhD., environmentalist and phytoestrogen researcher, states in the New Zealand Medical Journal (Vol. 113, 2/11/2000), "There is potential for certain individuals to consume levels of isoflavones in the range that could have goitrogenic effects. Most at risk appear to be infants fed soy formulas, followed by high soy users and those using isoflavone supplements." We have always been against soy for babies. Infants raised on soy milk show a high degree of thyroid autoimmune disease later in life.

If there is a weakness in the thyroid gland, soy can make it worse. Soy contains specific flavoins that have been clearly demonstrated as goitrogenic (anti-thyroid). Hashimoto's Disease (hypothyroid) indicates a need to eliminate soy from the diet.

It is now known that the phytoestrogens in soy have influenced the early onset of menstruation for girls as young as 8-9 years old.

We have found consistently that when people have a thyroid problem, they test negatively on soy. The Soy Online Service states that 30 mg. of soy isoflavones will have a negative impact on thyroid function.

In addition to these pros and cons, we have found that some people can metabolize fermented soy, such as miso, tempeh and soy sauce, but not unfermented soy such as tofu and soy milk.

Vegetarian Soy Menu Plans

These menus are to give you soy meal ideas.
It is best to eat soy only once or twice per day.

DAY 1

Breakfast   Vegetable breakfast link
Brown rice
Green salad

Lunch   Canadian bacon (soy) sandwich on sprouted flourless bread
Optional: egg-free mayonnaise, mustard, thinly sliced
cucumbers, lettuce, thinly sliced tomatoes
Soy milk

Dinner   Tofu slices fried over low heat in roasted sesame oil
Stir-fried vegetables (e.g., leeks, red bell peppers,
mushrooms, zucchini)

DAY 2

Breakfast   Tofu scramble (pg. 45)
Sprouted flourless toast
Green salad

Lunch   Tofu hot dogs
Sprouted flourless hot dog buns or sprouted flourless bagels
Optional: egg-free mayonnaise, mustard, horseradish
Celery sticks

Dinner   Tempeh
Brown, forbidden black, or basmati brown rice
Green beans
Tossed salad

DAY 3

Breakfast   Protein Drink *(pg. 40)*
Sprouted flourless toast
Raw green vegetable of your choice

Lunch   Black beans with brown rice
Salad

Dinner   Tofu turkey
Sprouted flourless bread stuffing
Asparagus
Tomato and cucumber slices

Other Breakfast Options

- Grilled soy cheese sandwich on sprouted flourless bread; mixed green salad
- Leftover stir-fry with brown rice
- Breakfast links sliced into brown rice; add okra

Other Lunch Options

- Miso soup with tofu cubes and chopped chives or scallions; rice crackers
- Sandwich made with thin slices of vegetarian meats
- Tofu Egg-free Egg Salad (pg. 91) sandwich on sprouted flourless bread

Other Dinner Options

- Tofu meat(less) balls with brown rice
- Tofu Spanish rice
- Tofu burgers

Happy, Healthy Children

*Alleviate Attention Deficit Disorder (ADD), Attention Deficit
Hyperactive Disorder (ADHD), irritable behavior, mood swings,
lethargy and allergies*

When children begin their day with sugared cereals, sugared toaster pastries, carbonated beverages, chocolate drinks, and refined flour, their bodies' vitamins and minerals become depleted. Refined foods are anti-vitamin and anti-mineral substances in their bodies. Children then lack the energy and ability to concentrate. Their nervous systems become overstimulated. The nervous system and digestive system are not capable of metabolizing foods without good nutrition.

Vitamin and mineral-fortified foods in reality are foods that have chemical nutrition made in laboratories. A child's body lacks the necessary enzymes to assimilate chemical supplements. These 'foodless' foods are more expensive in the long run.

Natural, whole foods can keep a child healthier and out of the doctor's office.

The specific foods that can keep your child healthy and happy are high-quality, whole, natural foods. Foods high in Vitamin B and mineral content are essential for proper brain and body development. These foods are listed in the Vitamin Chart (pgs. 140-141) and Mineral Chart (pg. 143) located in the Appendix.

Children's Menu Plan

Breakfast Eggs
Sprouted flourless whole grain toast
Whole grain cereals, such as oats, bear mush, cream of rice, or cream of buckwheat

Lunch See Lunches and Brown Bag Lunches *(pg. 34)*

Dinner See suggested Dinner list *(pg. 35)*

Snacks Encourage nutritious snacks, such as homemade cookies or cookies from the health food store that are sugar- and wheat-free
Whole grain crackers
Fruit Sorbet *(pg. 129)*
Fresh, raw fruits and vegetables
Raw nuts or Home-roasted Nuts *(pg. 70)*

Get your children involved in their own health by including them in the food preparation process. It will teach them, in their early years, the importance of taking time to make delicious, nutritious foods that can make a difference in their attitude toward themselves.

Quality time between you and your children is a loving ritual that can make a difference in who they are as individuals, ultimately making a difference on this planet.

Recipes

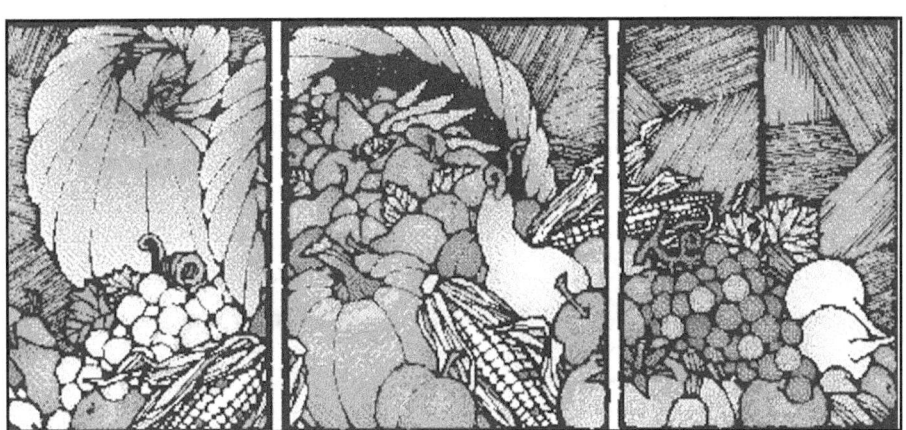

APPETIZERS / SNACKS

GOMASIO

1 cup organic sesame seeds, unhulled
1 teaspoon salt, sun-dried, noniodized

Put 1/4 cup sesame seeds into a dry skillet.
Cook over high heat, stirring often, until toasted.
This takes approximately 2 minutes.
Spread out on cookie sheet to completely cool.
Repeat with remaining sesame seeds.
Put 1/4 cup seeds at a time into blender.
Process for 5 seconds. **Do not completely chop seeds.**
Place blended seeds into bowl and stir in salt.
Place into a shaker jar with medium-size holes.
Sprinkle on toast, salads, or any food of your choice.

HOME-ROASTED NUTS

Spread nuts of your choice on a cookie sheet.
Roast for 30 minutes at 225°-250°.   *Yum!*

MUSHROOM PUREE

1/2 pound mushrooms
2 cloves garlic, chopped
2 ounces mineral bouillon *(found at health food stores)*
1 bunch garden cress or green's substitute, such as spinach
1/2 bunch parsley, minced
2 ounces extra virgin olive oil

Put all ingredients into blender.
Blend until smooth.

SALMON LOAF APPETIZER

3 tablespoons eggless mayonnaise
1 tablespoon lemon juice
2 teaspoons minced red onion
1 teaspoon horseradish, without vinegar
1/4 teaspoon sea salt
1 tablespoon minced parsley
1 1-pound can salmon
1/2 cup chopped pecans

Mix mayonnaise, lemon juice, onion, horseradish, sea salt and parsley.
Add salmon and mix well.
Shape into balls.
Roll in pecans.
Chill and reshape, if necessary.

TOFU DIP

1/2 pound tofu
1/3 cup tahini
Juice of 1 lemon
Sea salt and black ground pepper to taste

Put all ingredients into bowl.
Mash together with a fork and serve.
Use blender for a creamier dip.

Breads

SPELT BISCUITS

1/4 cup butter
1 teaspoon sugar
1 teaspoon sea salt
2 cups spelt flour
3 teaspoons baking powder
3/4 cup water

Pre-heat oven to 450°.
Cut butter into flour until it resembles coarse meal.
Add rest of dry ingredients.
Stir in water and mix lightly.
On flour-covered board, fold over and pat down 2-3 times.
Pat out and cut into biscuits. Place on greased cookie sheet and bake.
Bake in 450° oven for 10-12 minutes.

SPELT FRENCH BREAD

1 package yeast   3 cups spelt flour
1 cup warm water   1 teaspoon sun-dried sea salt

Pre-heat oven to 400°.
Put warm water into a bowl and sprinkle with yeast.
Let it sit a few minutes until dissolved.
Stir in flour and sea salt.
Mix until thoroughly blended.
Place on floured board and knead until dough is smooth and not sticky.
Additional flour may be needed.
Let rise for 30 minutes.
Punch down and shape into a long, thin loaf.
Let the dough rise again for 20 minutes.
For crisper bread, rub 1 tablespoon butter on top of bread before baking.
Bake at 400° for 20 minutes
or until the loaf sounds hollow when tapped.

ZUCCHINI BREAD

3 eggs
1 cup succanat
1/2 cup an organic, cold-pressed oil
3/4 cup unsweetened applesauce
1 Tbsp vanilla extract
3-1/2 cups flour
1 teaspoon sun-dried sea salt
1 teaspoon baking powder
1 teaspoon baking soda
1 teaspoon each cinnamon and nutmeg
2 cups grated zucchini
1 cup nuts *(optional)*

Pre-heat oven to 350°.
Beat eggs slightly.
Add succanat, oil, applesauce and vanilla.
Mix in flour, sea salt, baking powder, baking soda and spices.
Mix well.
Stir in zucchini and nuts.
Pour into 2 greased loaf pans.
Bake at 350° for approximately 50 minutes.

NOTE: A combination of oil and applesauce has less calories than using only oil, and makes the loaf very moist.

SOUPS

SIMPLE SOUP SUPPER

A bowl of homemade soup is the perfect meal any time of year.
Use one of the following recipes to create a Simple Soup Supper.

Just before serving, add a small amount of miso or tamari (if no salt restrictions.)
Serve with your choice of:

- Sprouted flourless whole wheat toast
- Spelt bread
- Whole grain bagel
- Belgian or Norwegian flat bread
- White or blue corn tortillas
- Whole wheat pita bread
- Rice with almond bread
- Bran bread
- Fruit-sweetened millet bread
- Sesame rice crackers

VEGETABLE STOCK

2 large onions, halved
4 carrots, peeled
1/2 cup Russian kale, chopped
1 clove garlic, halved
3 stalks celery, cut into 2-inch pieces
1 cup fresh parsley
8 cups water
4 tomatoes, quartered *(optional)*

Combine ingredients in soup pot.
Bring to boil.
Reduce heat to simmer.
Cover and cook 1 hour.
Let sit 30 minutes.
Strain and skim.

Stock may be frozen for later use.
Pour into 1-cup storage bags or freeze in ice cube trays.

Recipes

Soups For Carnivores
SPINACH AND FISH SOUP

2 onions, sliced
2 celery stalks, sliced
1/4 teaspoon ground mace
1/2 teaspoon fresh thyme (1/8 teaspoon dried)
1 bay leaf
5 cups fish stock or unsalted chicken stock
1 pound fillet from a firm, white-fleshed fish, such as grouper,
    haddock or pollock, skinned and cut into 1-inch chunks
2 tablespoons cream of buckwheat
1-1/2 pounds spinach, stemmed and washed

Put onions, celery, mace, thyme and bay leaf into a large pot.
Pour in 1 cup of stock and bring mixture to a boil.
Cover pot, reduce heat to maintain a strong simmer, and cook vegetables and seasonings for 30 minutes. Remove lid and increase heat to medium-high.
Cook mixture until liquid has evaporated and onions are lightly browned— about 10 minutes more.
Meanwhile, pour remaining 4 cups of stock into a large skillet over medium-high heat and bring to a simmer.
Add fish chunks and poach in the simmering stock until they are opaque and feel firm to the touch—about 3 minutes.
Remove fish pieces with a slotted spoon and set aside; reserve the poaching liquid.
Transfer 1 cup of poaching liquid to a small saucepan and bring to a boil.
Whisk in the cream of buckwheat and cook the liquid until it thickens— about 4 minutes.
Set liquid aside.
Pour remaining poaching liquid into pot containing the vegetables.
Stir in the spinach and cook it over medium-high heat until it wilts—about 4 minutes.
Puree spinach mixture with the buckwheat-thickened liquid in two batches in a blender or food processor. Return soup to the pot over medium heat.
Stir in fish pieces, and cook the soup for 2 minutes.
Serve immediately.

Suggested accompaniment: brown rice wafers.

GRACE'S TURKEY SOUP

Prepare Grace's Baked Turkey Thighs *(see page 108)*
2 cups brown rice, cooked
2 cups water

Remove onions from bottom of turkey thigh baking dish and place in blender with 2 cups water. Process for about one-half minute.
Cut cooked turkey into 1/2-inch pieces.
Add more herbs and spices to taste.
Add brown rice.
Cook 15-20 minutes.

CHICKEN AND LEEK SOUP

2 pieces of chicken on the bone
1 onion, chopped
2 stalks celery, sliced
3 cloves garlic, chopped
2 leeks, cleaned and sliced
2 carrots, sliced
3 tablespoons extra virgin olive oil
Italian seasoning
4 cups water
1 can organic chicken broth *(optional)*

Remove skin from chicken.
Heat oil in soup pot.
Cook chicken, onion, celery, garlic and leeks for about 10 minutes.
Add seasonings.
Add carrots and water.
Cook for 1 hour.
Remove meat from bone and return meat to soup.
Cook for 15 minutes.
For added flavor, add canned chicken broth.

Suggested accompaniment: rice cakes or rice crackers.

CHICKEN, BROWN RICE AND GREEN BEAN SOUP

1 piece chicken, breast or thigh, chopped
1 onion, chopped
1 stalk celery, sliced
2 cloves garlic, chopped
3/4 cup brown rice (brown basmati is best)
1/4 pound green beans
2 cups chicken broth
2 tablespoons extra virgin olive oil
3 cups water

Heat oil in soup pot. Add chicken, onion, celery and garlic.
Cook for 10 minutes.
Add rest of ingredients.
Cook for 1 hour.

Suggested accompaniment: spelt biscuits. (pg. 71)

Soups For Herbivores

CARROT SOUP

2 tablespoons extra virgin olive oil
1 pound carrots, cut into chunks
1 medium onion, chopped
2 stalks celery, sliced
2 cloves garlic, chopped
1/4 teaspoon dill
1 tablespoon parsley flakes
3-4 cups water

Heat olive oil in a Dutch oven.
Add carrots, onion, celery and garlic.
Cook for 8-10 minutes.
Add dill and parsley.
Add water and cook until carrots are soft—about 10 more minutes.

BLACK-EYED PEAS AND COLLARD GREEN SOUP

1 cup dried black-eyed peas
1 tablespoon cold-pressed safflower oil
3/4 cup onion, chopped
1 ounce Canadian bacon (soy), diced into 1/4-inch pieces
1 clove garlic, finely chopped
1 bay leaf
1/4 teaspoon crushed hot red-pepper flakes
5 cups unsalted vegetable stock or chicken stock
8 ounces collard greens, stalk removed, washed, coarsely
   chopped (about 4 cups)
2 teaspoons cider vinegar

Rinse peas under cold running water.
Put peas into a large, heavy pot and add enough cold water to cover them about 3 inches.
Discard any peas that float to the surface.
Cover pot, leaving lid ajar, and slowly bring to a boil over medium-low heat.
Boil peas for 2 minutes.
Turn off heat, cover, and let peas soak for at least one hour.
(Alternatively, soak peas in cold water overnight.)
Heat oil in a large, heavy-bottomed pot over medium heat.
Add onion and sauté, stirring occasionally, until translucent—about 4 minutes.
Add bacon (turkey or soy) and garlic.
Cook for 2 minutes, stirring frequently.
Drain peas and add to the heavy-bottomed pot along with bay leaf, red-pepper flakes and stock. Bring to a boil.
Reduce heat to maintain a simmer; partially cover pot.
Cook soup for 30 minutes, stirring gently several times.
Toss in collard greens, and cook until greens are soft and peas are tender —about 20 minutes.
Remove and discard bay leaf.
Stir in vinegar.
Serve the soup immediately.

Suggested accompaniment: spelt muffins or spelt biscuits (pg. 71).

NOTE: Mustard greens or kale may be substituted for collard greens; either of these vegetables will require 10-15 minutes less cooking time than the collard greens.

Recipes

HOT AND SOUR SOUP

6 cups unsalted chicken stock
1/4 cup rice vinegar
2 tablespoons Chinese black vinegar or balsamic vinegar
1-2 teaspoon chili paste with garlic or
   5-10 drops hot red-pepper sauce
1 tablespoon low-sodium soy sauce
1 tablespoon dry sherry
1 teaspoon finely chopped garlic
1-2 teaspoons finely chopped fresh ginger
1 carrot, julienne
6 dried shitake or Chinese black mushrooms, stemmed, the caps
   thinly sliced
   —cover with boiling water and soak 20 minutes
1/4 cup cloud-ear mushrooms *(optional)*, thinly sliced
   —cover with boiling water and soak 20 minutes
16 lily buds *(optional-see note below)*, trimmed, each bud tied
   into a knot—cover with boiling water and soak 5 minutes
3/4 cup bamboo shoots *(optional)*, rinse and julienne
2 tablespoons arrowroot powder mixed with 3 tablespoons water
8 ounces firm tofu, cut into thin strips
3 scallions, sliced diagonally into ovals

Heat stock in a large pot over medium-high heat.
Add vinegars, chili paste or hot red-pepper sauce, soy sauce, sherry, garlic, ginger, carrot and undrained shitake or Chinese black mushrooms.
If using, also add the cloud-ear mushrooms, lily buds (both undrained) and bamboo shoots.
Bring to a boil, then stir in arrowroot mixture.
Reduce heat and simmer, stirring until it thickens slightly—about 2-3 minutes.
Gently stir in tofu.

Ladle soup into bowls and garnish each serving with scallion slices.

NOTE: The lily buds called for are dried buds of common day lilies, available at Asian markets. They add unusual texture and flavor to the soup.

Homemade Vegetable Soup

2 tablespoons butter
3 cloves garlic, chopped
2 medium onions, thinly sliced
1/2 green cabbage, thinly sliced
4 stalks celery, sliced
5-6 carrots, cut into chunks
4 fresh beets, chopped (also use tops, if desired)
4 cups fresh tomatoes or home-canned tomatoes
4 cups homemade chicken broth
4 cups water
1/2 teaspoon dill seed or dill weed

In a soup pot, sauté onions and garlic in butter over low heat.
Add cabbage, celery, carrots and beets.
Sieve tomatoes and add to pot. Add chicken broth and water.
Add dill seed or dill weed.
Simmer 45 minutes.

Notice the house smells like a garden!

VEGETARIAN MINESTRONE

4 potatoes, cut into large dice
1 onion, diced
2 cloves garlic, chopped
2 stalks celery, sliced
2 carrots, diced
1 zucchini, peeled, diced
2-3 tomatoes (fresh tastes better than canned)
1 16-ounce can of organic beans;
     choose from navy, Great Northern, red kidney or garbanzo
1 cup rice noodles
Italian seasoning

Add all ingredients, except pasta, into soup pot.
Add 4 cups water.
Simmer until vegetables are soft and flavors are blended—about 20 minutes.
Add rice noodles and cook until noodles are al dente, approx. 20 minutes.
You can add some pizzazz by adding vegetable bouillon cubes.

PEARL BARLEY VEGETABLE SOUP

1/2 cup pearl barley, washed
8 cups water
1 cup sliced celery
1 cup diced carrots
1/2 cup sliced onion or leeks
1/2 red bell pepper, diced
3 teaspoons parsley, minced
2-1/2 tablespoons extra virgin olive oil
1 cup chard, kale or spinach, finely cut or chopped
1 teaspoon sweet basil
1 teaspoon oregano
1 teaspoon thyme

Start barley and water cooking in 2-quart pot.
Allow to cook 30 minutes before adding vegetables.
On medium-low heat in nonstick skillet, stir-fry the vegetables and herbs in olive oil for 5 minutes.
Cover and let them sweat for 3 minutes. Stir and cover again.
Turn heat to low for 3 minutes. Add vegetables to barley.
Continue cooking for another 30 minutes.

POTATO CORN CHOWDER

2 tablespoons extra virgin oil
1 onion, chopped
2 stalks celery, sliced
2 cloves garlic, chopped
2 pounds potatoes, cut into large dice
1/4 teaspoon dill
1 tablespoon parsley flakes
1/8 teaspoon cayenne pepper
1 package organic frozen corn
4 cups water

Heat oil in large skillet. Sauté onion, celery, garlic and potatoes.
Add dill, parsley and cayenne. Add water.
Cook 10-15 minutes, or until potatoes are soft.
Add more water if necessary, depending on potatoes.
Slightly blend soup for creamier texture, if desired.
Add corn just before serving.

VEGETABLE MILLET SOUP

1 ounce dry seaweed, nori or wakame
1/4 cup millet
1 stalk celery, finely chopped
1/2 red bell pepper, finely chopped
1 clove garlic, minced
1 cup green onion, finely chopped
1 carrot, finely chopped
5 cups vegetable stock
2 tablespoons dark *(flavored)* sesame oil
1 tablespoon tamari soy sauce
1-1/2 tablespoons lemon juice
Parsley, chopped for garnish

Put seaweed in small container and cover with cold water.
Soak for 3-4 minutes.
Drain liquid into a bowl.
Finely chop seaweed (easier to do with scissors).
Set both aside.

Heat oil in a soup pot over medium heat.
Add millet and sauté for 5-6 minutes, stirring often.
Add celery, bell pepper, seaweed, garlic and green onion.
Cook for another 7-8 minutes.
Add vegetable stock and seaweed water.
Bring soup to a boil.
Reduce heat to medium-low and cover pot.
Cook 30-40 minutes.
Add tamari and lemon juice. Stir well.

Pour into soup bowls and garnish with chopped parsley.

SALADS

Salads For Carnivores

EGG SALAD

4 hard-boiled eggs, chopped
2 tablespoons safflower mayonnaise
1/8 teaspoon organic mustard powder

Plus your choice of any or all of the following:
1 medium scallion, finely chopped
2 tablespoons celery, finely chopped
2 tablespoons red bell pepper, finely chopped
1 teaspoon pimento, finely chopped
6 Spanish olives, finely chopped

Mix all ingredients in a bowl.
Add sea salt and black ground pepper to taste.

GRILLED CHICKEN SALAD WITH THAI NOODLES

1 package Thai noodles
1 head Romaine lettuce
1 carrot, shredded
1 stalk celery, sliced
1/2 red cabbage, shredded
1 red onion, thinly sliced
1 cucumber, sliced
2 boneless, skinned chicken breasts

Cook Thai noodles as package directs.
Prepare a mixed salad with Romaine lettuce, carrots, celery, red cabbage, red onion and cucumber.
While the noodles cool, cook chicken on the grill.
Place salad on a platter, cover with Thai noodles and top with slices of grilled chicken.

SHRIMP AND GREEN BEAN SALAD

1 pound medium shrimp, shells left on
1-1/2 pounds green beans, trimmed and cut in half
1-1/2 teaspoons tarragon vinegar
1 tablespoon cold-pressed safflower oil
2 tablespoons fresh tarragon, chopped or 2 teaspoons dried
2 tablespoons chives, finely cut
1 tablespoon fresh parsley, chopped

Bring 8 cups of water to boil in a large saucepan.
Add beans and boil until just tender—about 6 minutes.
Drain beans and refresh them under cold running water.
Pat beans dry and transfer to a bowl. Set bowl aside.

Bring 4 cups of water to a simmer in the saucepan.
Add shrimp, cover pan, and simmer shrimp until they are opaque
—about 2-3 minutes.
Drain shrimp; when they are cool enough to handle, peel them (and, if you
like, devein them).
Add shrimp to beans.

To make the the marinade, in a small bowl, whisk together the tarragon
vinegar, oil, half of the tarragon, and 1 tablespoon of the chives.

Arrange the shrimp and beans on a serving platter; cover with the vinegar-
and-oil marinade.
Let the shrimp and beans marinate at room temperature for 30 minutes.
Near the end of marinating time, prepare dressing.

Whisk together parsley, the other half of the tarragon and the 1 tablespoon
of chives.
Pour dressing into a small serving bowl and serve it alongside the salad.

Suggested accompaniment: Whole-wheat pita bread

THAI LEMON-LIME SHRIMP SALAD

1 cup snow peas, raw
3 tablespoons fresh lemon juice
3 tablespoons fresh lime juice
2 shallots, thinly sliced
1-1/2 tablespoons cilantro or parsley, chopped
1 tablespoon fresh mint, chopped or 1 teaspoon dried
2 tablespoons fish sauce or low-sodium soy sauce
2 cloves garlic, finely chopped
1 small dried red chili pepper *(optional)* —soak in hot water 20
   minutes, drain, seed and chop
2 scallions, thinly sliced
1 pound medium shrimp, peeled, deveined if necessary, and
   halved lengthwise
2 heads of Boston lettuce or 4 heads of Bibb lettuce, washed
   and dried
4 mint sprigs

Put raw snow peas into a large bowl and toss with lemon and lime juices, shallots, cilantro or parsley, mint, fish sauce or soy sauce, garlic, chili pepper and scallions.

Bring 2 quarts water to a boil in a saucepan.
Add shrimp and cook until opaque—30 seconds to 1 minute.
Drain shrimp and transfer to the bowl.
Gently mix shrimp into the salad.
Cover bowl and refrigerate salad for at least 30 minutes.

Serve salad on lettuce leaves on individual plates, each portion garnished with a sprig of mint.

SLIMMING SEAFOOD SALAD

1 pound fish fillets, skinned (use any white fish, including
   trout)
1 cup boiling water
2 tablespoons fresh lemon juice
1/2 small onion, thinly sliced
1 sprig parsley, minced
1 teaspoon whole allspice
Cayenne pepper to taste
1/2 teaspoon seasoned salt
Salad greens
1 tomato, cut in wedges
1 cucumber, sliced
1 stalk celery, slice

Thaw fish if frozen.
Place fish in well-oiled frying pan.
Add lemon juice, onion, parsley and allspice. Pour in water.
Cover and simmer 5-10 minutes, until fish flakes easily with a fork.
Carefully remove fish, drain, and place in covered dish in refrigerator to chill.

Arrange salad greens on a plate.
Place tomato wedges, cucumber and celery slices around edge of greens.

Heap chilled fish in center.
Add seasoned salt and black ground pepper just before serving.

Suggested accompaniment: 1-2 tablespoons Oil Mix (pg. 11) or low-calorie organic salad dressing.

Salads For Herbivores

Avocado and Tomato Salad

3 avocados, diced
4 tomatoes, diced
6 cucumbers, diced
4 green onions, sliced
3 ears corn, uncooked, kernels cut off

Dressing
1 teaspoon lemon thyme
1/4 teaspoon rosemary
1/2 cup extra virgin olive oil

Whisk dressing ingredients.
Put all salad ingredients into bowl and toss gently.
Add dressing and toss again.

Bird's Nest Salad A La Sylvia

10 Romaine lettuce leaves
1 cup raw spinach
1 teaspoon minced parsley
1/4 cup alfalfa sprouts
6-8 cherry tomatoes
8-10 black olives, pitted
Shred lettuce and spinach. Toss gently with parsley.

Make a bed of the greens in a salad bowl and put a ring of sprouts around the inner rim of the bowl.
Place olives and tomatoes in the center.

Suggested accompaniment: nondairy dressing.

DIFFERENT POTATO SALAD

1 large boiled or steamed potato, grated
1 red onion, sliced
5 stalks celery, sliced
2 heads red or green leaf lettuce
1 head Bibb lettuce

Dressing
1 tablespoon mineral powder *(found at health food stores)*
1 teaspoon kelp
1/2 cup extra virgin olive oil

Toss salad ingredients.
Whisk dressing and pour over salad.

ROMAINE AND SPINACH SALAD

2 heads Romaine lettuce, shredded
1/2 bunch spinach, shredded
1/4 bunch parsley, chopped
4 stalks celery, sliced
1/2 red onion, sliced

Dressing
1 tablespoon mineral powder *(found at health food stores)*
1 teaspoon nutritional yeast
1 teaspoon kelp
1/2 cup extra virgin olive oil, or any other cold-pressed oil of
your choice

Whisk dressing ingredients.
Arrange greens and onion in salad bowls.
Pour dressing over salads.

ROMAINE SALAD WITH AVOCADOS

1 head Romaine lettuce, shredded
1 tablespoon parsley, chopped
1 large avocado, diced
1 small red onion, sliced
1 small cucumber, diced
1 medium tomato, cut in wedges
2 cloves garlic
1/8 teaspoon sweet basil
1/8 teaspoon marjoram
1/8 teaspoon cayenne pepper *(optional)*
Sea salt *(optional)*
Mineral broth *(found at health food stores or on the Internet)*
3-6 tablespoons extra virgin olive oil, or any other cold-pressed
    oil of your choice
1 teaspoon apple cider vinegar

Prepare the marinaded first.
Sea salt (if allowed) and mineral broth to taste.
Squeeze fresh garlic into salad bowl.
Add sea salt, pepper and seasonings.
Pour in vinegar and toss gently.
Marinate for at least 15 minutes.

Then add 3-6 tablespoons of oil to taste.
Let flavors blend.

Prepare the vegetables (chop, dice, slice, etc.)
Taste the marinade before adding vegetables, and adjust to your taste—this
often seems to vary even when using the same amounts. Also, the oil may
be mixed 2 parts cold-pressed oil to 1 part olive oil.

Add prepared lettuce, parsley, avocado, onion, cucumber and tomato.
Toss and serve.

RED AND WHITE BEAN SALAD

1/2 pound red kidney beans
1/2 pound Great Northern beans
1 small celeriac (Chinese celery), peeled and 1/2" cubed
1 small onion, thinly sliced
2 teaspoons finely chopped fresh ginger
1/2 cup rice vinegar
1 tablespoon chopped cilantro, mint or basil
1 large ripe tomato, diced
1-1/2 tablespoons safflower oil

Rinse kidney beans under cold running water. Put into a large pot with enough cold water to cover them by about 3 inches.
Rinse Great Northern beans under cold running water.
Put in a separate pot with enough cold water to cover them by about 3 inches. Discard any beans that float to surface.
Cover pots, leaving lids ajar, and slowly bring liquid in each to a boil.
Boil beans for 2 minutes, then turn off heat and soak the beans covered, for at least an hour.

(Alternatively, soak beans overnight in cold water.)
If beans absorb all of their soaking liquid, add enough water to cover them again by 3 inches.

Bring liquid in each pot to a boil, reduce heat to maintain a strong simmer, and cook beans until just tender—50 to 60 minutes.
While beans are cooking, peel celeriac and cut into 1/2-inch cubes.
Transfer cubes to a salad bowl and toss with onion, ginger and vinegar.
Set bowl aside at room temperature.

Drain cooked beans and rinse under cold running water.
Drain beans again.
Add to bowl tomato and oil. Then add cilantro, mint or basil.
Mix well.

Serve chilled or at room temperature.

BROCCOLI SALAD WITH OVEN-ROASTED MUSHROOMS

2 pounds mushrooms, wiped clean, stemmed
(Use your favorite mushrooms: white, portobello, shitake.)
4 large shallots, thinly sliced lengthwise
1/3 cup fresh lemon juice
2-1/2 tablespoons fresh thyme or 2 tablespoons dried
1 tablespoon cold-pressed safflower oil
2-1/2 pounds broccoli, stemmed and cut into florets
1 head of red or green leaf lettuce, washed and dried

Mustard Dressing
2 tablespoons grainy mustard
3 tablespoons balsamic vinegar
  or 2-1/2 tablespoons rice vinegar
1 teaspoon honey
1 tablespoon chopped fresh parsley
2 teaspoons chopped fresh oregano or 1/2 teaspoon dried
1 tablespoon safflower oil

Preheat oven to 450°.

Put mushrooms in a large baking dish.
Add shallots, lemon juice, thyme and oil; toss mixture to coat mushrooms.
Spread mushrooms into a single layer.
**Roast mushrooms until tender and most of the liquid has evaporated—
20-25 minutes.**
Remove mushrooms from oven and keep warm.

While mushrooms are cooking, make the dressing.
Combine mustard, vinegar, honey, parsley and oregano in a small bowl.
Whisking vigorously, pour in the tablespoon of oil in a thin, steady stream.
Continue whisking until dressing is well combined; set dressing aside.

Pour enough water into a saucepan to fill it about 1-inch deep.
Set a vegetable steamer in pan and bring water to a boil.
Put broccoli florets into steamer, cover pan, and steam broccoli until tender
but still crisp—about 4 minutes.
Add broccoli to dish with mushrooms.
Pour dressing over vegetables and toss the salad well.

Arrange salad on a bed of lettuce leaves; it may be served warm or chilled.

TOFU EGG-FREE EGG SALAD

1 12-ounce package firm silken tofu, diced
1/4 cup sweet red pepper, minced
3 tablespoons eggless mayonnaise
1 stalk celery, thinly sliced
1 tablespoon fresh Italian parsley, chopped
1 teaspoon yellow mustard
3 tablespoons pickle relish
1/2 teaspoon low-sodium soy sauce
1/4 teaspoon turmeric
1/4 teaspoon garlic powder

Combine all ingredients in a large bowl.
Mix well. Refrigerate for at least 30 minutes, or until well-chilled.

Sandwich suggestions:
4 organic whole wheat pita pockets or 8 sprouted flourless bread slices,
4 romaine lettuce leaves, and 4 tomato slices *(optional)*.

If using pita bread, cut the very top off each pita.
Open the pocket and line with tomatoes and lettuce.
Stuff with tofu filling.

VEGETABLES

ASPARAGUS IN CREPES

8 packaged crepes (made with spelt, or gluten-free flour)
3 tablespoons extra virgin olive oil
2 tablespoons water
1-1/2 pounds asparagus
2 red onions, chopped fine
2 red bell peppers, chopped fine
1/2 pound mushrooms, thinly sliced
2 tomatoes, chopped, hand-squeezed
1/2 pound black olives, pitted and halved
2 yellow squash, diced
2 zucchini, diced

Preheat oven to 450° for 10 minutes.
Put olive oil and water in a roasting pan.
Add the rest of the ingredients, except crepes.
Reduce oven to 300° and cook vegetables for 8-10 minutes.
Remove from oven and carefully lift out asparagus spears and place a few inside each crepe. Roll up crepes and place on a serving platter.
Cover with remaining vegetables and juice from pan.
Serve and enjoy.

CARROTS LIGHTLY

10 carrots, sliced
2 tablespoons mineral powder *(found at health food stores)*
1/4 teaspoon sweet basil
1 teaspoon cashew butter
1 teaspoon almond butter
1/2 cup raisins
Juice of 1 lemon
1/2 bunch parsley, chopped

Put carrots into steamer and sprinkle with mineral powder.
Add 1/4 cup water to pan and cover.
Steam for 5-8 minutes.
Mix nut butters together.
Mix in raisins, juice and herbs.
Toss with carrots.

CHOPPED EGGPLANT WITH PEAS

3 eggplants, cubed
1 pound peas
1/3 cup fresh sweet basil, chopped or 1-1/2 teaspoons dried
1 sweet potato, thinly sliced
4 tablespoons organic butter, sweet-cream, unsalted
1 teaspoon vegetable broth powder

Preheat oven to 450° for 10 minutes.
Place cubed eggplant in a covered roasting pan.
Reduce oven to 350° and bake eggplant for 10 minutes.
Open roasting pan, add peas and basil.
Cover again and bake for another 3-5 minutes.

While this is cooking, sauté sweet potato in butter.
Remove roasting pan from oven; spoon contents onto serving dish.
Top with sautéed sweet potato and sprinkle with powdered vegetable broth.
Serve hot.

MUSHROOMS AND PEAS

1 tablespoon butter-oil mix (pg. 11)
2 cloves garlic, finely minced
2 cups fresh mushrooms, chopped (portobellos are favorites)
1/4 teaspoon nonirradiated onion powder
1 package frozen baby peas, thawed
1/4 teaspoon sun-dried sea salt
1/4 teaspoon freshly ground pepper

Melt butter-oil mix in large, nonstick skillet over medium heat.
Add garlic and cook about 1 minute, or until it sizzles.
Add mushrooms.
Cook, stirring frequently—about 3 minutes.
Add onion powder.
Stir in peas and cook 3 minutes more, or until heated through.
Remove from heat and serve hot.
Add salt and pepper, or let guests add salt and pepper to their own taste.

SESAME STIR-FRIED ASPARAGUS

12 ounces fresh asparagus
1-1/2 tablespoon dark sesame oil
1/2 red bell pepper *(optional)*
1 clove garlic, thinly sliced *(optional)*

Break tough end off asparagus. Discard ends.
Cut each spear diagonally into 1-1/2-inch pieces.
Heat nonstick skillet over medium-high heat until drops of water sprinkled on skillet dance on surface.
Add oil. Tilt skillet to cover surface.
Add asparagus, bell pepper and garlic.
Cook, stirring constantly, 3-4 minutes or until asparagus turns bright green.
This goes well with any chicken, turkey, fish, lamb or beef dish.
Leftovers are great to use in a salad the next day.

STEAMED MIXED VEGETABLES

4 carrots, peeled and cut into chunks
1 onion, cut into wedges
1/2 pound green beans
2 potatoes, cut into quarters
2 cloves garlic, sliced
2 stalks broccoli, chopped
1 tablespoon dill
1 tablespoon fresh basil, chopped

In a steamer basket, place carrots, onion, green beans, potatoes, garlic and broccoli.
Sprinkle vegetables generously with dill and chopped fresh basil.
Steam until tender.

Suggested accompaniments: a mixed salad and French bread.

STIR-FRIED VEGETABLES

1 tablespoon extra virgin olive oil
2 carrots
1 celeriac (Chinese celery) or Jerusalem artichoke
1-2 parsnips
2 stalks celery
2 cloves garlic, squeezed
1 red onion, sliced
1 cup broccoli pieces
Seasoned salt
1 tablespoon sesame seeds or sesame salt
1 bunch parsley, chopped

Dice vegetables into 1-inch pieces.
Heat oil in large frying pan. Add carrots, celeriac and parsnips.
Cook for about 5 minutes.
Add celery, onion and garlic.
Cover and cook over medium heat for 5-10 minutes.
Stir often with a wooden spatula to keep from sticking. Vegetables should still be crisp.
Sprinkle with sea salt, sesame seeds and parsley.

NOTES:
Parsley is a good blood purifier, as well as a natural breath freshener.

Garlic is a panacea for many ills, and is excellent for keeping blood pressure down

----

THERMOS FLASK LUNCH

1/4 cup yellow mung dhal (type of dried pea), washed well
1/4 cup basmati brown rice (wash well)
1-1/2 cups fresh vegetables, cut to size that will fit into thermos
Spices to taste (sea salt, pepper, cumin, ginger, turmeric, etc.)
1 tablespoon ghee (clarified butter)
2 cups water

The best ghee is made with organic unsalted cultured butter by heating on low heat until milk solids seperate and the oil floats.

Skim off the milk solids. The butter is now clarified.
In a pot, gently fry ground spices in the ghee for a few seconds.
Add mung dhal, rice and chopped vegetables.
Cover well with water and bring to a boil.
Boil only 2 minutes.
Without wasting time, pour into a 1 liter thermos flask.
Use a spoon to get the vegetables in more easily.
Screw on the lid quickly and leave the thermos closed for about 4 hours.

The meal will cook and be ready to eat by lunchtime.

VEGETABLE TORTILLAS

1/4 cabbage, thinly sliced
1 small onion, thinly sliced
2 stalks celery, thinly sliced
1 small carrot, grated
2 cloves garlic, minced
1 teaspoon parsley
1 teaspoon dill
2 tablespoons extra virgin olive oil
4-6 tortillas of your body's choice (corn, spelt or wheat)
Grated cheese (soy, rice or almond)
Fresh organic tomatoes, diced

Combine cabbage, onions, celery and carrots.
Sauté in olive oil for 3-5 minutes.
Add garlic, parsley and dill.
Cook until vegetables are tender.

Serve on tortillas with grated cheese and diced organic tomatoes.

For extra flavor use some tamari, soy sauce or salsa.

NOTE: For non-vegetarians, replace carrots with 1/4 cup cooked, minced chicken or shrimp.

Recipes

MAIN DISHES

Main Dishes For Carnivores

BEEF

BEEF PAPRIKA

1 1-1/4-pound boneless sirloin steak, trimmed of fat and cut
  into 4 pieces
2-1/2 tablespoons paprika, preferably Hungarian
2 tablespoons organic flour (whole wheat or spelt)
1 tablespoon organic, cold-pressed safflower oil
1 onion, cut into 1-inch cubes
1 green pepper, seeded, deribbed and cut into 1-inch squares
1 garlic clove, finely chopped
1-1/2 cups unsalted vegetable stock or unsalted chicken stock
1/4 pound mushrooms, wiped clean, cut in half if large

Combine 2 tablespoons of paprika, and flour on a plate.
Dredge steak pieces, coating each one evenly.
Reserve remaining flour-paprika mixture.
Heat 1 teaspoon oil in a nonstick skillet over medium-high heat.
Sear meat and set aside.
Wipe pan clean with a paper towel; heat remaining teaspoons oil in pan.
Add onion, green pepper and garlic; sauté, stirring occasionally, until
onions are translucent—about 5 minutes.
Add remaining flour-paprika mixture, then whisk in the stock.
Add meat and bring stock to a simmer.
Cover pan and simmer beef and vegetables for 1 hour and 15 minutes.
Stir in mushrooms and remaining 1/2 tablespoon of paprika.
Cook mixture, covered, for 15 minutes longer.

Serve the beef surrounded by the vegetables and covered with the sauce.

Suggested accompaniments: rice noodles and broccoli.

ORGANIC BEEF TENDERLOIN ROAST WITH SPINACH SAUCE AND ALMONDS

1-3/4 pounds beef tenderloin roast, fat trimmed off
2 tablespoons cold-prssed safflower oil or extra virgin olive oil
2 tablespoons slivered almonds
3 tablespoons finely chopped shallots
1 cup dry white wine
1/2 pound fresh spinach, stemmed and washed
1/4 cup unsweetened soy milk or almond milk
1/8 teaspoon nutmeg
1/8 sea salt and/or freshly ground pepper to taste

Preheat oven to 325°.

Heat 1 tablespoon of oil in a large, nonstick skillet over high heat.

Sear meat on all sides until brown (2-3 minutes total time).

Transfer tenderloin to roasting pan. Do not wash skillet.

Finish cooking meat in oven —about 45 minutes or until meat thermometer registers medium-well.

Heat a small, heavy-bottomed skillet over medium heat.

Add slivered almonds.

Toast almonds, stirring constantly, until lightly browned—about 2-3 minutes.

Remove from skillet and set aside.

To make sauce:

Heat remaining 1 tablespoon of oil in the large skillet used for browning meat.

Add shallots and cook until translucent—about 2 minutes.

Pour in wine. Simmer until about 1/3 cup remains—about 6-8 minutes.

Remove roast from oven. Let sit 10 minutes while sauce is being prepared.

Add spinach to shallot-wine mixture. Reduce heat to low.

Cover and cook until spinach has wilted—about 1-2 minutes.

Stir in milk and nutmeg. Return heat to simmer.

When simmer begins, pour into blender or food processor.

Add 1/8 teaspoon sea salt and some freshly ground pepper.

Process until pureed.

Carve roast into 12 slices and arrange on warmed platter.

Spoon some sauce over slices of meat and sprinkle with almonds.

Serve remaining sauce separately.

Remember to serve sun-dried, noniodized sea salt and fresh ground pepper.

BEEF TENDERLOIN ROAST WITH SPINACH AND SPROUTS

1 2-1/2-pound beef tenderloin roast, trimmed of fat
2 tablespoons toasted sesame seeds
4 tablespoons low-sodium soy sauce
3 tablespoons rice vinegar or cider vinegar
1/4 teaspoon powdered stevia
1 tablespoon cold-pressed safflower oil
3/4 pound fresh spinach, washed, stemmed and sliced into
    1/2-inch wide strips
4 cups bean sprouts

To make marinade, puree 1 tablespoon sesame seeds, 3 tablespoons soy sauce, 2 tablespoons vinegar and stevia in a blender.

Put tenderloin into a shallow dish and pour marinade over it.
Let stand for 2 hours at room temperature, turning meat occasionally.

Preheat oven to 325°.
Drain tenderloin and pat dry with paper towels.
Discard marinade.
Pour oil into a large ovenproof skillet set over high heat.
When oil is hot, sear meat until well-browned on all sides—3-5 minutes.
Place skillet in oven.

For medium-rare meat, roast tenderloin for 40-45 minutes, or until a meat thermometer inserted in center registers 140°.

Remove meat from oven and let it rest while preparing the garnish.

Heat a large skillet or wok over medium heat.
Add spinach strips and cook, stirring constantly, until liquid has evaporated —about 2-3 minutes.
Stir in tomatoes and sprouts.
Cook vegetables until heated through—about 3-4 minutes more.
Remove pan from heat and stir in remaining soy sauce and vinegar.

Cut tenderloin into 16 slices and arrange on a platter.
Surround beef slices with spinach-and-sprout garnish.
Sprinkle remaining sesame seeds over the garnish.

Suggested accompaniment: brown rice or quinoa tossed with finely chopped scallion greens.

STIR-FRIED BEEF WITH GINGER

1 pound top-round steak, trimmed of fat and sliced into 2 inch
long thin strips
1/2 tablespoon cold-pressed peanut* oil
1 bunch watercress, trimmed, washed and dried

Ginger Marinade
1 2-inch piece of fresh ginger, peeled and finely chopped
1 tablespoon chili paste or 1 tablespoon hot red-pepper flakes
1/4 cup dry sherry
1/4 cup unsalted chicken stock
2 tablespoons arrowroot powder for thickening
1/4 teaspoon stevia

Cucumber Salad
2 cucumbers, seeded and cut into thick strips
1/4 cup rice vinegar
1 tablespoon dark sesame oil

Combine marinade ingredients in a bowl.
Add beef and toss well; cover bowl and marinate meat for 1 hour at room
temperature.

Combine cucumbers, vinegar and sesame oil in a bowl.
Refrigerate the salad.

When marinating time is up, drain beef, reserving marinade.
Heat oil in a large, nonstick skillet or wok over high heat.
Add beef and stir fry until well browned—about 2 minutes.
Add reserved marinade; stir constantly until sauce thickens—about 1
minute.
Add watercress and toss mixture quickly.

*Serve the stir-fried beef and watercress immediately, accompanied by the
chilled cucumber salad.*

Suggested accompaniment: brown rice with sweet red peppers.

* *If allergic to peanuts, use a different cold-pressed oil.*

Recipes

LAMB

LAMB STEW WITH RED PEPPER AND OKRA

1-1/4 pounds lean lamb (from the leg or loin), trimmed of fat
  and cut into 1-inch pieces
1/4 cup organic flour (whole wheat or spelt)
2 tablespoons paprika
1 tablespoon cold-pressed safflower oil
1 onion, finely chopped
1-1/2 cups unsalted vegetable stock or unsalted chicken stock
2 tablespoons cider vinegar
1 teaspoon Dijon mustard
8 drops hot red-pepper sauce *(optional)*
1 garlic clove, finely chopped
1 sweet red pepper, seeded, deribbed and cut into 1-inch squares
1/2 pound okra, trimmed, cut in half if large
1/2 cup brown rice

Combine flour and paprika in a large bowl.
Toss lamb pieces in flour mixture.
Remove meat from bowl, shaking off any excess flour, and set aside.

Heat oil in an ovenproof casserole over medium-high heat.
Add lamb and onion.
Cook, stirring continuously, until onion is translucent and meat is
browned—2-3 minutes.
Stir in stock, vinegar, mustard, hot red-pepper sauce, garlic, sweet red
pepper and okra.
Bring mixture to a simmer.
Reduce heat to low and simmer stew, stirring every now and then, until
meat is tender—30-40 minutes.

Meanwhile, bring 1 cup water to a boil in a saucepan.
Add rice, tightly cover pan, and reduce heat to medium-low.
Cook rice until all liquid has been absorbed—about 20 minutes.

When meat is tender, stir the cooked rice into the stew and serve at once.

Suggested accompaniment: mixed green salad.

CHICKEN, BEEF OR LAMB

STIR-FRIED MEAT AND GREEN BEANS

Use your choice of:
1-1/4 pounds lean lamb (from the leg or loin), trimmed of fat
  and cut into thin strips,
  1 pound thin strips of top-round steak, or
  1-1/4 pounds thin chicken strips
1 cup unsalted vegetable stock or unsalted chicken stock
2 tablespoons brandy
1 teaspoon low-sodium soy sauce
1-1/2 tablespoons rice vinegar
1 shallot, chopped
1/2 pound green beans, trimmed and cut in half on the diagonal
1-1/2 tablespoons cold-pressed safflower or extra virgin olive oil
2-3 small dried red chili peppers, finely chopped, or 1 teaspoon
  hot red-pepper flakes *(optional)*
2 teaspoons fresh ginger, peeled and finely chopped
4 garlic cloves, finely chopped

Heat stock in small saucepan over medium heat.
Add brandy, soy sauce, vinegar and shallot.
Simmer mixture until it is reduced to about 1/4 cup—15-20 minutes.
Set sauce aside.

While sauce simmers, steam green beans until tender but still crisp—about
3-4 minutes.
Remove beans from pan and refresh under cold running water.
Then set beans aside.

Heat oil in a large nonstick skillet or well-seasoned wok over medium-high
heat.
Add chili peppers or red-pepper flakes, ginger and garlic.
Stir-fry for 1 minute.
Add beans and meat and continue stir-frying until meat is lightly browned
and just cooked through—about 2 minutes.
Pour sauce over the meat and beans, stir well, and cook for 30 seconds more.

Serve at once over brown rice or brown rice spaghetti.

Recipes

CHICKEN

CHICKEN PAPRIKA

2 tablespoons extra virgin olive oil
3 organic chicken breasts, skinless, cut into bite-sized pieces
1 large onion, sliced
2 cloves garlic, chopped
1 stalk celery, sliced
1 tablespoon paprika
1 can organic chicken broth

Heat oil in large skillet.
Add chicken, onion, garlic and celery.
Stir-fry until chicken begins to brown.
Add paprika.
Cook for at least 20 minutes, stirring frequently.
Add chicken broth; cook 15 minutes more.

Serve over pasta or rice.

EASY CURRIED CHICKEN

2 tablespoons extra virgin olive oil
2 organic chicken breasts, skinless, cut into strips
1 onion, chopped
1 stalk celery, sliced
3 cloves garlic, chopped
2 tablespoons curry powder, or to taste
2 cups organic chicken broth

Heat olive oil in large skillet.
Add chicken strips, onion, celery, garlic and curry powder.
Sauté until onion is transparent.
Add chicken broth. Simmer until chicken is thoroughly cooked
    —about 20 minutes.
For thicker broth, use 2 teaspoons arrowroot powder or cornstarch
dissolved in 2 tablespoons cold water.
Stir in 1/2 cup broth from pot.
Stir until smooth and add back to pot.

Serve over brown rice.

CROCKED CHICKEN AND BROWN RICE

2 tablespoons organic, cold-pressed cooking oil
1 small onion, chopped
1 large clove garlic, chopped
1 stalk celery, sliced
2 organic chicken breasts, skinless, cut into bite-size pieces
8 green beans, sliced diagonally
1 cup brown rice
1 cup organic chicken broth
3 cups water

Heat oil in large skillet.
Add onion, garlic and celery.
Cook 3 minutes.
Add chicken and cook until chicken begins to brown.
Add green beans.
Continue cooking for another 5 minutes.
Stir in rice.

Pour into crock pot.
Add broth and water.
Set on low heat.
Cook until rice is well done.

NOTE: **If you cook this all afternoon, the rice will be done in time for dinner.**

BAKED CHICKEN AND TOFU

1 2- to 3-pound organic frying chicken, in serving-sized pieces
1 pound tofu, cut in 1-inch cubes
1/2 pound green beans, whole or cut in half
2 onions, cut in wedges
1 cup snow peas
3 tablespoons organic, cold-pressed cooking oil
1/4 cup soy sauce
Red chili, garlic powder or your favorite herbs

Pre-heat oven to 350°.
Mix soy sauce, seasonings and oil.
Gently toss tofu in oil mixture, then remove and set aside.
Toss remaining ingredients in the oil mixture.
Add tofu, mix, then place in a large baking pan.
Bake at 350° for at least 1 hour, or until chicken is done.

CHICKEN STEW

1 organic chicken, cut into serving-size pieces
3 tablespoons organic, cold-pressed cooking oil
1 medium leek, chopped
2 cloves garlic, chopped
2 stalks celery, sliced
1 tablespoon basil
1 tablespoon parsley
1 tablespoon thyme
2 large carrots, diced
1 cup chard or kale, finely cut
1/2 pound green beans, cut in half
1 cup organic chicken broth
1 cup water

Heat oil in large pot and sauté onion, garlic, celery and herbs to season.
Add chicken, broth and water. Simmer for 15 minutes.
Add carrots, chard or kale, and green beans.
Simmer until vegetables are tender—about 15 minutes more.

Suggested accompaniments: brown rice and salad.

TOFU AND EGG OMELET

1 pound tofu, mashed
3 tablespoons organic, cold-pressed cooking oil
4 eggs
4 scallions, chopped
1/2 red bell pepper, chopped
1/2 teaspoon thyme
1/2 teaspoon dill
1/4 cup soy sauce
1/2 teaspoon garlic powder
Black pepper to taste
1/2 cup grated cheese (rice Parmesan)

Heat the oil in a large skillet.
Crack eggs into a bowl and beat lightly.
Stir in scallions, bell pepper, thyme, dill, soy sauce and garlic powder.
Pour eggs into skillet.
Cook over low heat for 10 minutes.

Black pepper to taste—add after cooking
Top with cheese.
Place under broiler until cheese is browned.

Suggested accompaniment: sprouted flourless tortillas, sprouted flourless toast or white corn tortillas.

Recipes

TURKEY

GRACE'S BAKED TURKEY THIGHS

2 organic turkey thighs, skinned
1/2 lemon or lime, juiced
1 medium onion, sliced
1/4 cup water
1 tablespoon extra virgin olive oil or other cold-pressed cooking oil
Seasoned salt
Sweet basil, marjoram, Fines herbs or Italian herbs
2 tablespoons butter

Preheat oven to 500°.
Place turkey thighs in a dish and sprinkle with juice.
Let stand for 10 minutes.
Line bottom of baking dish with onion slices and add 1/4 cup water.
Grease thighs lightly with oil and sprinkle with herbs.
Place on top of onions in dish.
Top each thigh with 1 tablespoon butter.
Place dish into oven and immediately reduce temperature to 350°.
Bake for 40-45 minutes.

TURKEY MEAT LOAF

1 pound ground turkey
1 egg
1/2 cup chopped onion
1 stalk celery, chopped
1 cup cooked brown rice
1/2 teaspoon dill
1/2 teaspoon basil

Pre-heat oven to 350°.
Combine all ingredients.
Shape into loaf and bake in 350° oven for at least 30 minutes.

Experiment by adding different flavors such as grated carrots or zucchini.

STUFFED CABBAGES OR PEPPERS

Filling

2 tablespoons extra virgin olive oil
1 small onion, chopped
1 pound organic ground turkey
2 stalks celery, sliced
1 large clove garlic, chopped
1 teaspoon parsley
2 cups cooked brown basmati rice

Heat oil in large skillet.
Add onion, celery and garlic.
Add turkey, cook and stir until meat is browned.
Cook meat thoroughly.
Add cooked rice and parsley.

Let cool while preparing cabbage leaves or peppers.

Stuffed Cabbages

8-10 cabbage leaves, steamed until soft

Pre-heat oven to 350°.

Place about 1/4 cup filling onto center of each cabbage leaf and roll up, tucking ends under.
Place rolls into oiled casserole dish.
Add 1/3 cup water.

Cover and bake at 350° for 30-40 minutes.

Stuffed Peppers

6 red or green bell peppers, washed and seeded

Pre-heat oven to 350°.

Fill peppers with turkey and rice mixture.
Place into oiled casserole dish.
Add 1/3 cup water.

Cover and bake at 350° for 30-40 minutes.

GROUND TURKEY MEATBALLS WITH GRAVY

1 pound ground turkey
1 egg or egg substitute
1/2 cup cooked brown rice
1 stalk celery, sliced very thin
1 small onion, chopped
2 cloves garlic, minced
4 tablespoons extra virgin olive oil
2-3 tablespoons arrowroot powder
1/4 cup organic chicken broth

Combine ground turkey, egg, brown rice, celery, onion and garlic.
Mix well and shape into meatballs.
Heat olive oil in large skillet and add meatballs; brown on all sides.
Add chicken-flavored broth and a little water.
Cook in broth until meatballs are completely done—about 20 minutes.
Add arrowroot to thicken gravy.

Make more gravy, if you like, by adding more broth and arrowroot.

Serve over spelt pasta, quinoa or rice.
Suggested accompaniment: steamed vegetables.

FISH

OCEAN PERCH CREOLE

1-1/2 teaspoons butter
1 small onion, chopped
1 green pepper, seeded, deribbed, chopped
1 garlic clove, finely chopped
1-1/2 pounds ripe tomatoes, peeled, seeded, chopped
    or one 12-ounce can of unsalted, whole tomatoes, drained
  and coarsely chopped
1/2 cup fish stock or water
1 cup okra, thinly sliced
3 tablespoons Dijon mustard
2 tablespoons paprika
1/2 pound small shrimp, peeled and deveined
1/2 cup spelt flour
2 tablespoons cold-pressed safflower oil
1-1/4 pounds ocean perch fillets (or red snapper or striped bass),
    skin left on, cut into 6 equal pieces

To prepare the sauce:
Melt butter in a saucepan over medium heat. Add onion and green pepper.
Cook, stirring occasionally, until onion becomes transparent and begins to
turn golden—4-5 minutes.
Add garlic and cook, stirring, for 30 seconds.
Stir in tomatoes, stock or water, okra, mustard and paprika.
Bring mixture to a boil, reduce heat to medium-low and simmer for 5 minutes.
Stir in shrimp and cook sauce for 1 minute more.
Set saucepan aside.

Rinse fillets under cold running water and pat dry with paper towels.
Place fish in a paper bag with spelt flour and shake bag to coat the fillets.
Heat oil in skillet over medium-high heat.
Sauté fillets in the oil until they are opaque all the way through—
approximately 2 minutes per side.

Reheat sauce and pour it into a serving platter.
Lay the fillets on top of the sauce.
Suggested accompaniment: brown basmati rice or quinoa.

Recipes

FISH STEW

1-1/2 pounds mussels, scrubbed and debearded
1/2 pound squid, cleaned and skinned
1/2 pound medium shrimp, peeled and deveined
1 onion, chopped
1 cup dry white wine
2 ripe tomatoes, peeled, seeded and chopped
1 whole garlic bulb, cloves peeled and thinly sliced
1/4 teaspoon ground turmeric
1/4 teaspoon ground cumin
1/4 teaspoon ground coriander
1/8 teaspoon ground allspice
1/8 teaspoon ground cloves
1/8 teaspoon ground cardamom

Put mussels in a deep pot with onion and wine.
Cover pot tightly and cook over medium-high heat until they open
—about 5 minutes.
Discard any mussels that remain closed.
Let mussels cool, then remove them from their shells and set aside.
Strain the mussel cooking liquid into a bowl.

Let it stand for 2-3 minutes to allow any sand to settle out.
Slowly pour most of the liquid into a large, heavy-bottomed skillet, leaving
sand behind.
Add tomatoes, garlic and spices to skillet.
Bring liquid to a boil, then reduce heat to medium-low and simmer mixture
until garlic is tender —about 5 minutes.

Meanwhile, prepare squid.
Slit the pouches up one side and lay them flat on the work surface.
Use a sharp knife to score a crosshatch pattern on the inside of each pouch.
Cut scored pouches into 1-1/2-inch squares.
Chop the tentacles into small pieces.
Add squid to the liquid simmering in the skillet.
Cover skillet and cook mixture until squid pieces have curled up
—about 1 minute.
Add the shrimp, cover the pot and continue cooking until shrimp are
opaque—about 1 minute more.
Finally, add the mussels and cook the stew for 1 minute to heat mussels
through.
Serve at once.

Suggested accompaniment: quinoa with almonds.

GRILLED DILLED SALMON

1 pound salmon steaks
2 medium lemons, juiced
2 teaspoons dill
1 stick organic butter, sweet-cream, unsalted
1 tablespoon tamari

Melt butter in small saucepan.
Add lemon juice, dill and tamari.
Place salmon steaks into casserole dish and top with butter sauce.
Cover and refrigerate for a couple hours.
Put foil (bright, shiny side up) on grill and fold up the edges to preserve the tasty juices.
Place salmon on the foil.
Grill until tender and done
—about 5-10 minutes depending on the thickness of the steaks.

Planked Salmon Steaks

1-1/2 pounds salmon steak, thawed if frozen
2 tablespoons butter, melted
1 lemon, juiced
1 small onion, thinly sliced
1/2 teaspoon seasoned salt
1/2 teaspoon paprika
Parsley and lemon for garnish

Pre-heat oven to 350°.
Parsley sprigs and lemon slices for garnish
Place fish in a single layer on a preheated, oiled wooden plank or a well-greased broil-and-serve platter.
Combine butter, lemon juice, onion and seasonings. Pour over fish.
Bake at 350° for 25 minutes or until fish flakes easily with a fork.
Garnish with parsley and lemon.

Suggested accompaniment: 2-3 cups of a combination of two or more hot, cooked vegetables: asparagus, broccoli spears, green beans, mushrooms, sweet peas or tiny, whole onions.
Do not add corn, Brussels sprouts or cauliflower.

OVEN-STEAMED ROCKFISH

2 tablespoons dry sherry
2 teaspoons arrowroot
1 3-pound whole rockfish (or black sea bass or ocean perch),
    cleaned and scaled
1 2-inch piece of fresh ginger, peeled and julienned
4 scallions, trimmed and cut lengthwise
1/4 cup cilantro or parsley leaves, loosely packed
2 tablespoons low-sodium soy sauce
1 tablespoon Chinese black vinegar or balsamic vinegar

Preheat oven to 450°.

Combine sherry and arrowroot in a small bowl.
Rinse fish under cold running water and pat dry with paper towels.
Cut 4 or 5 slashes on each side of fish.
Rub the sherry marinade over fish, inside and out, working some into the slashes.
Place fish on the bright, shiny side of a large piece of aluminum foil and let it marinate for at least 15 minutes.

Insert a strip of ginger and a piece of scallion into each of the slashes on the fish.
Place remaining ginger, cilantro or parsley, and scallions in the body cavity.
Lay a few cilantro or parsley leaves on the outside of the fish; put remaining leaves in the cavity.

Combine soy sauce, vinegar and pour mixture over fish.
Fold foil over the fish and crimp the edges to seal package tightly.
Set foil package on a baking sheet and bake the fish until flesh is opaque and feels firm to the touch—about 25 minutes.

Carefully transfer fish to a warmed serving platter.
Pour over the fish any liquid that has collected in the foil during baking.
Serve immediately.

Suggested accompaniments: stir-fried green beans and water chestnuts and steamed brown rice.

SPICY SNAPPER WITH HOT SALSA

Use your choice of:
4 snapper fillets
4 catfish fillets
4 halibut fillets
4 bass fillets
1/4 cup fresh lime juice
2 tablespoons organic oil: extra virgin olive oil or cold-pressed afflower oil
1 cup unsalted white baked tortilla chips, finely crushed
1 teaspoon chili powder
1/4 teaspoon ground cumin
1 cup salsa
1/4 cup fresh cilantro, chopped

Preheat oven to 450°.
Lightly oil a cookie sheet.
Cut each fillet in half. Rinse in cold water and pat dry with paper towels.
Mix the lime juice and oil in a shallow dish.

In another dish, combine chips, chili powder and cumin.
Dip fish into the lime-oil mix, then press into the seasoned crumbs to coat.
Place on prepared baking sheet in a single layer.
Sprinkle with any remaining crumbs.

**Bake about 10 minutes, or until the coating is crisp
and the fish flakes when tested with a fork.**

Warm salsa in small saucepan over medium heat.
Spoon salsa over fish and sprinkle with cilantro.
Add sea salt and freshly ground black pepper at the table.

STRIPED BASS WITH MUSHROOMS ON A BED OF SPINACH

12 ounces mushrooms, wiped clean and sliced
1 small lemon, juiced
1 pound fresh spinach, washed and stemmed
  or 10 ounces frozen spinach, thawed
1 tablespoon cold-pressed safflower oil
1 onion, finely chopped
1/8 teaspoon grated nutmeg
1 pound striped bass fillets (or black sea bass, red snapper or rockfish),
  skin left on

Put mushrooms in a saucepan with lemon juice.
Pour in enough water to cover, then bring to a boil.
Reduce heat to medium and simmer until mushrooms are tender
  —about 5 minutes.
Set pan aside.

Put fresh spinach, with water still clinging to its leaves, in a large pot over medium heat.
Cover pot and steam spinach until leaves are wilted—2-3 minutes. (Frozen spinach needs no cooking.)
Squeeze moisture from spinach and chop it coarsely.
Heat oil in a large, heavy-bottomed skillet over medium heat.
Add onion and cook until it is translucent—about 4 minutes.
Drain mushrooms and add to skillet, stir in spinach and cook for 2 minutes.
Season mixture with nutmeg, then spread it evenly in the bottom of a flame-proof baking dish.

Preheat broiler.

Rinse the fillets under cold running water and pat dry with paper towels.
Lay fillets skin side up on vegetable mixture.

**Broil the fish until the flesh feels firm to the touch and skin is crisp
  —about 5 minutes.**

Serve immediately.

Suggested accompaniment: sautéed sliced turnips.

TROUT A LA VIVIAN

1/2 pound whole trout
1 teaspoon extra virgin olive oil or cold-pressed oil of your choice
1/4 teaspoon fresh garlic, minced
1/4 teaspoon seasoned salt
10 allspice berries
1 teaspoon lemon juice
2 teaspoons chopped parsley

Sprinkle inside of trout with seasoned salt, lemon juice, parsley and garlic.
Brush outside with oil.
Place in skillet.
Surround trout with allspice berries.
Add 1/2 cup water to skillet.
Cover and steam for 10 minutes.

Serve and enjoy while steaming hot.

SEAFOOD

SAUTÉED SHRIMP WITH SHERRY AND CHILIES

1 lb. shrimp, peeled and deveined, shells reserved
1 whole garlic bulb, cloves separated and peeled
4 dried red chili peppers (use caution when handling these)
1 teaspoon fresh rosemary, minced or 1/2 teaspoon dried
   or 1/2 teaspoon fennel seeds
1/3 cup dry sherry
1 red pepper, seeded, deribbed and julienne
1 scallion, trimmed, julienned
1 tablespoon unsalted butter

Put shrimp shells in a saucepan with garlic, chili peppers, rosemary or fennel seeds, in 1 quart of water.
Bring water to a boil, then reduce heat to medium-low and simmer the mixture for 30 minutes.
Strain the poaching liquid, discard solids and return liquid to saucepan.
Boil the liquid rapidly until only about 1-1/2 cups remain—5-10 minutes.
Pour in sherry and bring liquid to a simmer.
Poach the shrimp until they are opaque—about 1 minute.
Remove shrimp with a slotted spoon and set them aside.
Boil remaining poaching liquid until only 2-3 tablespoons remain
   —about 5 minutes.
Add the red pepper, reduce heat to medium and cook for 2 minutes.
Return shrimp to saucepan.
Add the scallion and butter; stir until butter has melted and shrimp are warm.
Serve immediately.

Suggested accompaniment: steamed brown rice.

SHRIMP WITH GINGER

1-1/4 lbs. medium shrimp, peeled and deveined, shells reserved
1-inch piece of fresh ginger, peeled, thinly sliced
1-1/2 cups dry white wine
1 pound dried black beans, soaked for at least 8 hours and drained
2 onions, chopped
4 garlic cloves, 2 crushed and 2 very thinly sliced
1 cinnamon stick, broken into 3-4 pieces
1 tablespoon grated lemon zest
1 tablespoon extra virgin olive oil
1/2 teaspoon ground cinnamon
1 tablespoon peeled, chopped fresh ginger
1 teaspoon fresh lemon juice
3 scallions, trimmed and thinly sliced

Put shrimp shells in a large saucepan.
Add the ginger slices, 1 cup of wine and 2 cups of water.
Bring mixture to a boil. Reduce heat to medium and cook until liquid is reduced by half—about 30 minutes.
Strain stock into a bowl, pressing down on shells to extract any liquid.
Set bowl aside.
While shells are cooking, put drained beans in a large, heavy-bottomed saucepan along with onions, crushed garlic cloves and the pieces of cinnamon stick.
Pour in enough water to cover beans by about 1-1/2 inches and boil the beans for 10 minutes. Skim off foam and reduce heat to low.
Add shrimp stock and lemon zest, and simmer mixture until beans are tender but not mushy and a thick sauce results—1-1/2 to 2 hours.
Remove the cinnamon-stick pieces and discard.
About 5 minutes before beans finish cooking, pour the oil into a large, heavy-bottomed skillet over medium-high heat.
When oil is hot, add the shrimp.
Add the chopped ginger, garlic and the ground cinnamon.
Sauté the shrimp, stirring frequently for 3 minutes.
Pour lemon juice and remaining 1/2 cup of wine into the skillet; continue cooking mixture, stirring frequently, until shrimp are opaque and liquid is reduced to a glaze—about 2-3 minutes more.
Stir in scallions.
Pour the beans onto a serving platter and top with the shrimp mixture.
Serve immediately.

Suggested accompaniment: crisp green salad.

NOTE: Speed up this recipe by using canned organic black beans.

VEGETARIAN

TOFU-MUSHROOM BAKE

1 pound tofu, cut into 8 slices
1/2 cup organic, cold-pressed cooking oil
1 large onion, thinly sliced
1/2 pound mushrooms, sliced
6 tablespoons flour (spelt, rice or oat)
1/2 cup baked rice wafers, crushed
1/4 cup soy sauce
2 cups water
1/4 teaspoon thyme
1 teaspoon onion powder
1 teaspoon garlic powder
1 teaspoon cumin
Pinch of sage
1/2 to 1 teaspoon red chili powder

Pre-heat oven to 350°.
Mix 2 tablespoons flour, rice wafers, thyme, onion powder, garlic powder, cumin and sage.
Bread each slice of tofu by pushing each side into flour-spice mixture twice.
Pour 2 tablespoons oil into baking pan and add tofu slices.
Bake the slices at 350° for 15 minutes.

Meanwhile, heat 2 tablespoons oil in skillet.
Cook onions until clear and fragrant.
Add mushrooms and cook until soft.
Remove from pan.
Add 2 tablespoons oil to skillet and heat.
Add 4 tablespoons flour and red chili powder.
Cook until fragrant and browned.
Mix soy sauce and water. Slowly add to flour, mixing well.
Stir in onions and mushrooms.

Meanwhile, turn tofu slices in baking pan, add remaining 2 tablespoons oil and continue baking.
Tofu slices should be browned on both sides about the same time the gravy has simmered enough to thicken.
Place tofu slices on brown rice and top with gravy.

SPELT PASTA AND SPINACH FEAST

1 box spelt pasta
1/2 cup onion, chopped
2 cloves garlic, chopped
2 tablespoons extra virgin olive oil
2 cups spinach, washed and chopped
1 teaspoon fresh basil leaves, chopped
1/2 teaspoon dill seeds
1/4 teaspoon thyme or Italian seasoning

Cook spelt pasta.
While pasta cooks, sauté onions and garlic in olive oil.
Add spinach, basil and dill.
Sauté for a few more minutes.
Add oregano and thyme or Italian seasoning.
Mix pasta with spinach sauce.

Suggested accompaniments: fresh green salad and spelt French bread.

LOST TOMATO PASTA SAUCE

2 medium zucchini or yellow crookneck squash, washed and
sliced lengthwise
1 medium red bell pepper, cored, seeded and sliced lengthwise
into 4 pieces
2 stalks celery, cut diagonally into 3 pieces each
1 large clove garlic, peeled
1 small red onion, quartered
1 small portobello mushroom, cut into 6 to 8 1/4-inch slices
(optional)
2 teaspoons fresh chopped basil (1 teaspoon dried)
1 teaspoon fresh oregano (1/2 teaspoon dried)
1 teaspoon fresh chopped parsley (1/2 teaspoon dried)
1 tablespoon extra virgin olive oil

The sauce may be cooked in skillet or in oven.

Heat oil in large skillet.
Add all vegetable ingredients and sauté for about 10 minutes,
OR
Place all vegetables on oiled cookie sheet.
Brush each piece with olive oil.
Roast 10-15 minutes or until zucchini is light brown.

Put into blender or food processor.
Add and blend spices into sauce.

*Serve hot over brown rice **or** buckwheat, rice or spelt spaghetti.*

QUICKIE PETITE PIZZA

Pre-heat oven to 350°.
1 organic sprouted flourless bread
1 Lost Tomato Paste Sauce
1 Your choice of toppings (olives, spinach, onions, etc.)
2 slices rice or soy cheese

Toast slice of organic sprouted flourless bread until medium-brown.
Spread with sauce, top with 2 slices soy or rice cheese.
Add any favorite toppings.
Bake at 350° until cheese melts.

Enjoy with salad or soup.

LOST TOMATO PIZZA

Pizza Dough

1 package yeast	1 cup warm water
2-1/2 cups spelt flour	1 teaspoon sea salt

Put warm water into a bowl and sprinkle with yeast.
Let sit a few minutes until dissolved.
Stir in flour and sea salt. Mix well.
Cover and let dough rest for 20 minutes.
Spread dough onto greased cookie sheet.
Add toppings of your choice.
Place into 400° oven and bake until lightly browned.

You can try adding Italian spices to the dough, such as basil, oregano and some garlic powder.

SOY BEAN LOAF

1 pound organic soy beans, washed
1/2 pound walnuts, chopped
2 slices homemade bread, made into crumbs
6 zucchini, diced
1/4 pound mushrooms, chopped
1/2 pound asparagus, chopped
4 tablespoons butter
1 tablespoon mineral powder *(found at health food stores)*
3 ears corn, uncooked, kernels cut off
2 tablespoons extra virgin olive oil
1 tablespoon water

Put soy beans in a large cooking pot and cover with water.
Soak overnight, or at least 12 hours.
After soaking, cook beans in same water for 20-30 minutes.
Drain well, and chop so beans are coarse and crunchy. Add walnuts and bread crumbs and mix well. Set bean mixture aside.
Preheat oven to 450°.
Sauté zucchini, asparagus and mushrooms in butter, olive oil and 1 tablespoon water. Cook for 5-7 minutes in an open skillet.
Add mineral powder.

Mix together sautéed vegetables with soy beans and nut mixture.
Form into a loaf and put into baking pan.
Reduce oven to 350° and bake for 7-10 minutes.
Remove loaf from oven and top with corn kernels.
Serve hot.

TOFU CURRY

2 pounds tofu, mashed
1 large onion, thinly sliced
2-3 cloves garlic, minced
2 tablespoons oil *(dark sesame oil works best)*
1/4 cup catsup, unsweetened
1 cup water
1/4 cup raisins *(optional)*
2 tablespoons chicken or vegetable broth

Spice Mixture
1/2 teaspoon cloves
2 tablespoons curry powder
1-1/2 teaspoon ginger powder
1 teaspoon sea salt
3/4 teaspoon cinnamon
3/4 teaspoon garlic powder

Heat oil in a large skillet.
Add garlic and onion.
Sauté until they begin to brown.
Reduce heat to low, add catsup and spices.
Cook for 2 minutes, stirring constantly.
Mix in remaining ingredients.
Bring to boil.
Reduce heat and simmer, covered, for 10 minutes, stirring once.

Good additions to sprinkle into the Curry: chopped cilantro, green peppers, cashews, or coconut.

Suggested accompaniments: brown rice, quinoa or millet.

STIR-FRY

Basic instructions for Stir Fry Recipes.

Cook vegetable combinations for stir-fries on medium heat, added in the order listed.

You may add liquid aminos, and/or tamari sauce.

Add freshly ground pepper before serving.

Garlic and onions are always optional.

Suggested oils are safflower, extra virgin olive, dark sesame or any other GOOD oil.

SESAME TOFU STIR-FRY

1 pound very firm tofu, drained and gently press-dried on towel
2 tablespoons dark *(flavored)* sesame oil
1 small onion, thinly sliced
8 shitake mushrooms
1 small red bell pepper, cut into thin strips
1 large green bell pepper, cut into thin strips
1 tablespoon sake or white wine
1 tablespoon soy sauce
1 teaspoon grated ginger root
1 tablespoon sesame seeds
2 tablespoons water
1/2 tablespoon arrowroot powder dissolved in 1 tablespoon water

Cut tofu crosswise into pieces the shape of French fries.
Heat oil in wok or skillet over medium heat.
Add onion and mushrooms.
Stir and toss for 1 minute.
Reduce heat to medium-low.
Add bell peppers.
Cook about 1 minute.
Add tofu and sesame seeds.
Cook another minute.
Reduce heat to low.
Add sake or wine, soy sauce, ginger and water.
Simmer 3-4 minutes.
Stir in dissolved arrowroot and mix well.
Simmer 30 seconds.

---

3 GREAT STIR-FRY COMBINATIONS TO TRY
See page 125 for Basic Instruction for Preparing these 3 Stir-Fry Combinations.

STIR-FRY #1

1-3 cloves garlic, minced
1/2 cup onion, sliced
2 teaspoons sweet basil
2 teaspoons rosemary
2 teaspoons ginger powder or dill weed
1/4 cup celery, sliced
1/4 cup green pepper, sliced
2 cups green cabbage, sliced
1 cup broccoli florets, cut into small pieces
1/2 cup jicama, sliced—added last to cook for a short time.

STIR-FRY #2

1-3 cloves garlic, minced
1/2 cup onion, sliced
2 teaspoons sweet basil
1 teaspoon Fines herbs
1/4 cup fresh parsley, finely minced
2 cups zucchini, sliced diagonally
1 cup Chinese cabbage, shredded
1 4-ounce can water chestnuts, quartered *(optional)*
1/4 teaspoon anise seed powder
1/4 cup green pepper, diced
1/4 cup celery, diced
1 small yam, diced
2 cups green cabbage, shredded
1/2 cup radishes and/or jicama, diced addes last to cook for short time.

STIR-FRY #3

The best of East and West stir-fry for those who cannot or should not eat beans and 'love' Mexican food:

1-3 cloves garlic, minced
1/4 cup onion, sliced
1 tablespoon fresh parsley, finely minced
2 tablespoons chili powder
1 teaspoon cumin powder
1/4 cup green, yellow or red bell pepper, diced
1/4 cup celery, sliced
1-1/2 cups green beans, sliced
1/4 cup fresh or frozen peas
Picante sauce
Roll into preheated corn or flour tortillas

NOTES:

- *Never* **cook salt or pepper as heating alters chemistry and the molecular structure, making them indigestible and harmful.**

- **Nuts can be added to any stir-fry except for the one with yams.**

- **Bean sprouts can be added just before serving**

Suggested accompaniment for all Stir-Fry recipes:
brown or brown basamati rice.

SWEETS AND SWEET IDEAS

BAKED APPLES #1

4 apples, Gala or Fuji (preferably organic)
1/2 cup raisins
1 teaspoon cinnamon

Pre-heat oven to 350°.
Wash apples and cut in half.
Top each half with raisins and cinnamon.
Wrap in foil. Bake at 350° for about 1 hour.

BAKED APPLES #2

4 apples, Gala or Fuji (organic please)
1 organic lemon
1/2 cup organic raisins, chopped coarsely
1/4 cup toasted pecans *(optional)*
2 tablespoons pure maple syrup
1 tablespoon cognac *(optional)*
1 teaspoon cinnamon
1/4 teaspoon ground cloves
1-1/2 teaspoons arrowroot powder
1-1/2 cups fresh orange juice

Preheat oven to 350°.
Using a paring knife or corer, make a 1-inch diameter hole in each apple.
Place the apples right side up in a 9-inch x 9-inch baking dish.
Grate the lemon rind into a medium bowl.
Cut lemon in half and squeeze juice into the bowl. Discard the lemon.
Stir in raisins, pecans *(optional)*, maple syrup, cognac *(optional)*, cinnamon and ground cloves.
Mix well and spoon into apples.
Place arrowroot powder in a small bowl.
Add orange juice and stir until smooth.
Pour around apples.
Bake at 350° for 50-60 minutes, or until softened.
Baste apples occasionally with the pan juices.

Serve warm.

STEWED APPLES

1-2 apples, peeled and cut into chunks
1/2 to 1 cup water
Cinnamon to taste

Cook apples in water until tender.
Add cinnamon and enjoy.

FRESH FROZEN PEACH DESSERT

1 cup peaches
1/2 teaspoon lemon juice
1/4 teaspoon cinnamon

Put all ingredients into blender and process until smooth.
Pour into a loaf pan.
Place dish in freezer.

This peach blend is refreshing, easy to make, and a wonderful sorbet.

FRUIT SORBET
Organic fruit is the very best

8 ripe pears, peeled, cored, quartered
1/2 cup frozen apple juice concentrate
2 tablespoons fresh lemon juice
2 cups sliced strawberries

Combine pears, apple juice and lemon juice in a food processor or blender.
Process until smooth.
Pour into an airtight container and freeze until solid. Usually about 2 hours.
Just before serving, remove the sorbet from freezer.
Break into chunks and reblend until smooth and light.

Serve topped with the strawberries.

Makes about 8 servings.

FRUIT CRISP DESSERT

2-3 cups fruit, fresh or frozen (thawed)
2 tablespoons succanat, or pure maple or rice syrup
1 cup spelt flour
1/4 cup organic, cold-pressed cooking oil

Preheat oven to 375°.

Lightly oil a 9-inch x 9-inch baking dish.
Place fruit into prepared baking dish.
In a bowl, combine oil and flour to make the crust.
Crumble crust over fruit.

Bake for about 25 minutes.

NOTE: If fruit is not very juicy, such as apple, add a little fruit juice to the mixture.

PEACH-BLUEBERRY CRISP

Filling
2 pounds ripe peaches, peeled, pitted and cut into 1/2-inch
    slices
2 cups blueberries
2 tablespoons pure maple syrup
2 tablespoons organic whole grain pastry flour (wheat, gluten-
    free or spelt)
1 tablespoon lemon juice
1/3 cup apricot or peach nectar
1/2 teaspoon coriander powder

Topping
1/2 cup organic whole grain pastry flour (wheat or spelt)
1/4 cup Rice Spoonfuls dry cereal
1/2 teaspoon cinnamon
3 tablespoons butter

Preheat oven to 375°.

Lightly oil a 9-inch x 9-inch pan.
In a large bowl, stir together all filling ingredients.
Pour into prepared baking dish.
In a medium bowl, stir together all topping ingredients.
Cut the butter into topping until mixture resembles coarse meal.
Sprinkle over the fruit.

Bake 45-50 minutes, or until the topping is lightly browned.

Let cool 10 minutes, then serve.

PECAN PUDDING

1 cup organic cornmeal

3/4 cup milk: soy, almond or rice drink

3 eggs or egg replacer plus 1-1/2 teaspoons lecithin granules for 'egg yolk'

1/2 cup succanat sugar

1/4 cup molasses

1/4 teaspoon baking soda

1/2 cup organic butter, sweet-cream, unsalted

1/2 cup raw pecans, chopped

1/4 cup organic whole grain pastry flour (spelt, gluten-free or wheat)

3 teaspoons baking powder

2 teaspoons cinnamon

1 teaspoon sea salt

1/8 teaspoon nutmeg

Preheat oven to 325°.

Lightly oil 1-1/2-quart casserole.

Combine 1/4 cup milk with 1/4 cup cornmeal.

Bring remaining milk to boil.

Gradually add cornmeal mix.

Stir constantly.

Return to boil and cook for 3 minutes.

Combine hot cornmeal and remaining ingredients.

Pour into casserole.

Bake for 1 hour and 10 minutes.

Suggested accompaniment: REAL organic whipped cream.

DATE NUT PUDDING

1 cup organic flour (spelt, gluten-free or whole wheat pastry)
1/2 cup succanat
1/2 cup chopped dates
1/2 cup water
1 teaspoon baking powder
Pinch of sea salt
1/2 cup pecans

Topping
1/2 cup succanat
1/4 cup molasse
1-1/4 cups boiling water
1 teaspoon vanilla
1 teaspoon butter

Preheat oven to 350°.
Lightly oil 9-inch x 9-inch pan.
Mix all ingredients except topping.
Pour into prepared pan.
Spread pecans over batter.
Mix topping and pour over batter.
Bake for 30 minutes.

CAROB CAKE

1/2 cup organic butter, sweet-cream, unsalted
1/2 cup carob powder
1-1/2 cups spelt flour
1/2 cup soy yogurt
1 teaspoon baking soda
3/4 cup molasses
1/2 cup hot water
1 teaspoon cinnamon

Preheat oven to 375°.
Lightly oil a 9-inch x 9-inch pan.
Stir together dry ingredients.
Add wet ingredients and blend well.
Pour into prepared pan.
Bake for 20-25 minutes.

HONEY CAROB CAKE

3 eggs
1 cup honey
3/4 cup carob powder
1 teaspoon pure almond extract
1 cup walnuts
1 cup yogurt
1/2 cup oil
1/2 teaspoon sea salt
1-1/2 cups organic pastry flour (spelt, gluten-free or whole
    wheat pastry)
2 teaspoons baking soda

Preheat oven to 375°.

Lightly oil two 9-inch x 9-inch pans.
Place everything except flour and baking soda in blender and blend until smooth.
Add flour and baking soda.
Blend quickly.
Pour into prepared pans.

Bake for 30 minutes.

Cool 10-15 minutes before taking out of pan.

CARROT PIE

2-1/2 cups carrots, cooked and drained
1/2 cup succanat sugar
1 egg or egg replacer plus 1-1/2 teaspoons lecithin granules for
    'egg yolk'
1 teaspoon sea salt
1/2 teaspoon cinnamon
1/2 teaspoon ginger powder
1/2 teaspoon nutmeg powder
1-3/4 cups milk: plain soy or almond
9-inch pie shell, or make crustless

Preheat oven to 450°.

Stir ingredients together.
Pour into pie shell.

Bake 10 minutes.
Then reduce heat to 300° and bake another 50 minutes.

Recipes

PUMPKIN SQUARES

2/3 cup butter

1 cup succanat

1 16-ounce can pumpkin (or equivalent fresh)

3 eggs or egg replacer plus 1-1/2 teaspoon lecithin granules for 'egg yolk'

2 cups flour (spelt, gluten-free or whole wheat pastry)

2 teaspoons pumpkin pie spice

2 teaspoons baking powder

1/2 teaspoon baking soda

Preheat oven to 350°.

Lightly oil a 10-inch x 15-inch jelly roll pan.

Stir together wet ingredients.

Stir in dry ingredients.

Pour into prepared pan.

Bake for 35-40 minutes.

RASPBERRY BARS

2 cups organic whole wheat pastry flour

1-1/2 cups brown sugar

or 3/4 cup succanat plus 1/4 cup molasses

1 teaspoon baking soda

1 cup organic butter, sweet-cream, unsalted

3/4 cup raspberry jam, fruit-sweetened

Preheat oven to 350°.

Lightly oil a 9-inch x 13-inch pan.

Mix all ingredients, except jam.

Blend until crumbly.

Sprinkle half into prepared pan.

Pat down and cover with jam.

Place remaining crumb mix on top.

Bake 30-45 minutes.

SUNNY OAT COOKIES

1/2 cup nut butter (almond, sunflower, hazelnut, or cashew)
1/4 teaspoon sea salt
1-1/2 cups oats
1/2 cup raw sunflower seeds
Few drops stevia

Preheat oven to 350°.

Lightly oil a cookie sheet.
Mix all ingredients.
Shape into balls.
Place onto cookie sheet and press with flat-bottomed glass dipped in flour.
Bake for about 12 minutes.

Recipe makes 1-2 dozen cookies.

Appendix

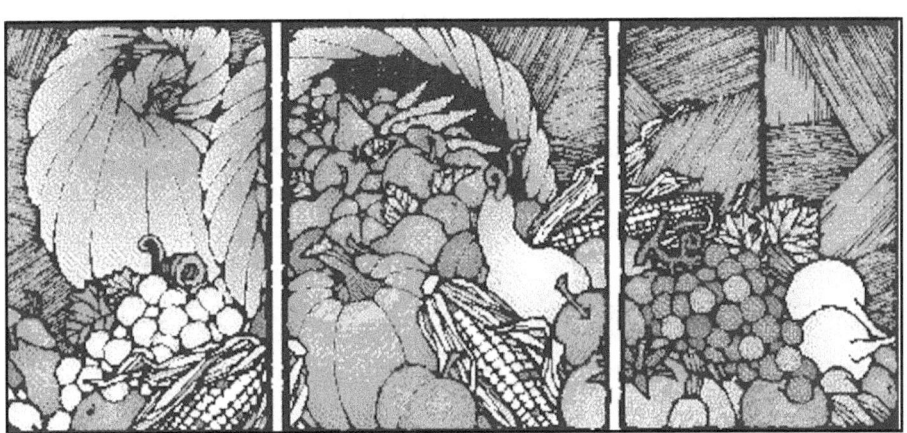

SUBSTITUTION LIST

**Many favorite recipes can be prepared more healthily
by using substitutes.**

**An additional benefit is that usually,
but not always,
the substitute is lower in calories.**

This chart can help with such substitutions.

Baking Base . . . .**Use**
Butter or margarine . . . . . . .Granulated lecithin

Beverages . . . .**Use**
Coffee . . . . .Grain beverages, green tea
Soda pop . . . . .Carbonated mineral water; add
. . . . .fruit juice or food grade essential oils
. . . . .to create your own soda flavors

Bread Crumbs . . . .**Use**
White bread . . . . .Wheat germ, rice bran, oat bran, whole
grain bread, brown rice flour bread

Dairy Products . . . .**Use**
Cottage cheese . . . . .Tofu
Ice cream . . . . .Organic bananas, tofu (blend then freeze)
Milk . . . . .Almond milk, soy, hemp or rice drink
Milk, Cheese . . . . .Cashews, blended butter, soy or rice cheese

---

Eggs . . . .**Use**
. . . . .Egg Replacer*, Tofu

Leavening . . . .**Use**
Baking powder . . . . .Non-aluminum baking powder

Protein and Extender . .**Use**
Meat . . . . .Tofu, Tempeh
Total vegetable protein (TVP)
Textured tofu

Note: When using "egg replacement" in a recipe, the amount of the lecithin granules used for the same amount of eggs is dependent upon the amount of flour in the recipe.

Pasta Noodles . . . . .Use
Semolina or Wheat . . . . .Brown rice, brown rice pasta, spelt pasta,
. . . . .buckwheat noodles, mung bean threads

Salad Dressing . . . . . . .Use
Oil . . . . .Tahini
Vinegar . . . . .Lemon juice
Mayonnaise . . . . .Tofu

Seasonings . . . . .Use
Animal/chicken broth . . . . . .Vegetable broth, liquid aminos
Chili powder . . . . .Cumin, curry
Cinnamon . . . . .Coriander
Packaged seasoning . . . . . . .Organic chicken seasoning
Soy sauce . . . . .Liquid aminos

Sweeteners . . . . .Use
Chocolate . . . . .Carob
Sugar . . . . .Apple juice, apple sauce, barley malt, dates,
date sugar, fresh or dried fruit, fruit juice
concentrate, kiwi sugar, grape juice, honey,
maple syrup, stevia, succanat sugar
Sugar syrup for canning . . . .Pineapple juice

Thickeners . . . . .Use
Jell-O . . . . .Agar, vegan gelatin
Wheat flour or cornstarch . . .Arrowroot, cornstarch, potato starch,
tapioca
Eggs . . . . .Egg replacer

Appendix

Vitamin Chart

ITS NAME	ITS FUNCTION	FOOD SOURCES
Vitamin A Retinol, Carotene	Helps maintain healthy tissues, necessary for good eyesight	Eggs, fruits and vegetables, especially green and yellow vegetables, fish, alfalfa
Vitamin B Complex*	Helps maintain energy levels, aids metabolism, and promotes muscle tone	Nuts, wheat germ, whole grains, plain yogurt, alfalfa
Vitamin B1 Thiamin	Helps build healthy blood, aids circulation and digestion	Blackstrap molasses, yeast, brown rice, organic meat and poultry, nuts and seeds, alfalfa
Vitamin B5 Pantothenic acid	Helps build antibodies, antihista-mine action, aids to reduce stress	All vegetables, eggs, fish, nuts, whole grains, alfalfa
Vitamin B6 Pyridoxine HCL	Aids in weight control, helps build antibodies to fight infection and disease	Avocados, bananas, blackstrap molasses, green leafy vegetables, nuts, whole grains, alfalfa
Vitamin B12 Cyano-cobalamin	Helps build healthy body cells and a healthy nervous system	Eggs, fish, sea vegetables
Vitamin B15 Panagamic Acid	Aids metabolism, improves functions of glands and nervous system	Brown rice, seeds, whole grains
Vitamin C Ascorbic acid	Antioxidant, anti-stress, aids digestion, anti-inflammatory, aids collagen production, helps build strong bones and teeth, promotes healing, red blood cell formation	All fresh fruits and vegetables, especially oranges, broccoli and peppers
Vitamin D Calciferol, Viosterol, Ergosterol	Helps build strong bones and teeth, aids heart action, maintains healthy nervous system, aids blood clotting	Egg yolks, salmon, tuna, sunshine, alfalfa
Vitamin E Tocopherols	Helps retard the aging process, aids fertility, antioxidant, helps reduce cholesterol, maintains capillary wall strength, maintains muscles and nerves, aids circulation	Butter, dark green vegetables, eggs, fruit, nuts, vegetable oils, wheat germ, brown rice, alfalfa

*B Complex = B1/Thiamin, riboflavin/B2, niacin, B4, B5 panto-thenic acid, pyridoxine/B6, biotin, folic acid and cyanocobala-min/B12, choline and inositol

Vitamin Chart

ITS NAME	ITS FUNCTION	FOOD SOURCES
Vitamin F **Fatty acids**	Helps prevent artery hardening, aids in blood clotting, helps maintain blood pressure, aids glandular activity	Vegetable oils, wheat germ, sunflower seeds
Vitamin K **Menadione**	Formation of blood clotting factor prothrombin	Alfalfa, leafy green vegetables, sea vegetables, yogurt, egg yolks, safflower oil, soy oil, fish liver oils
Biotin	Aids in building healthy cells	Egg yolks, legumes (peas and beans), nuts, alfalfa
Bioflavonoids	Anti-inflammatory, helps build blood vessel walls, helps heal bruises, good for cold and flu prevention and recovery, maintains strong capillary walls	Fruits (especially skins and pulp)
Choline	Helps prevent gallstone formation, aids in building a healthy nervous system	Egg yolks, legumes, wheat germ, soy lecithin, alfalfa
Folic acid	Aids in healthy cell growth, circulation, formation of HCL (hydrochloric acid) needed for digestion, important for expectant mothers	Red and green vegetables, cabbage family, citrus fruits, salmon, alfalfa
Inositol	Helps retard artery hardening, aids in cholesterol reduction, promotes hair and nail growth	Blackstrap molasses, citrus fruits, meat, nuts, vegetables, whole grains, alfalfa
Niacin	Aids circulation, cholesterol reduction, histamine activator (allergies), helps with metabolism, helps with production of sex hormones	Eggs, meat, poultry, fish, nuts, whole grains, sea vegetables, alfalfa
PABA **Para-amino-** **benzoic acid**	Helps build healthy blood cells, aids metabolism	Blackstrap molasses, bran, eggs, brown rice, wheat germ, alfalfa

Food Combining Chart

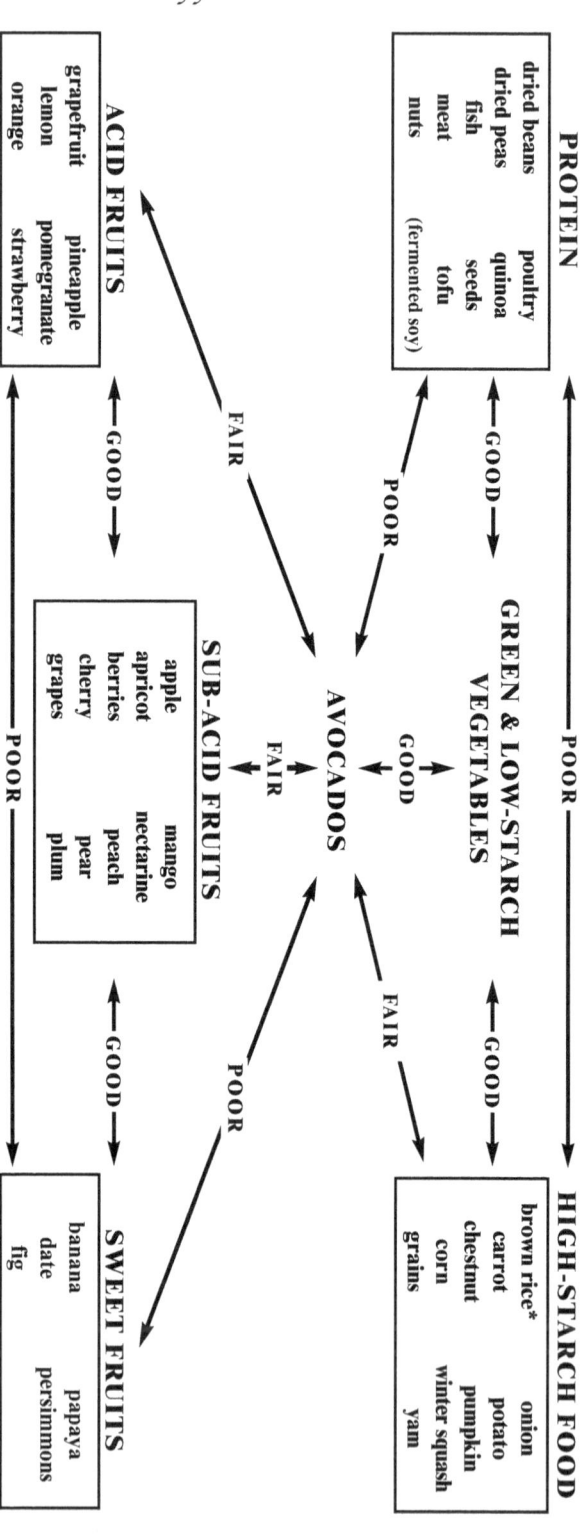

PROTEIN

dried beans	poultry
dried peas	quinoa
fish	seeds
meat	tofu
nuts	(fermented soy)

ACID FRUITS

grapefruit	pineapple
lemon	pomegranate
orange	strawberry

GREEN & LOW-STARCH VEGETABLES

AVOCADOS

SUB-ACID FRUITS

apple	mango
apricot	nectarine
berries	peach
cherry	pear
grapes	plum

HIGH-STARCH FOOD

brown rice*	onion
carrot	potato
chestnut	pumpkin
corn	winter squash
grains	yam

SWEET FRUITS

banana	papaya
date	persimmons
fig	

POOR — FAIR — GOOD — POOR

*Brown rice is an exception to the poor High-Starch/Protein relationship; it digests well with animal and vegetable proteins.

Eat only one concentrated protein food at a meal. • Tomatoes may be combined with low-starch vegetables and nuts or avocados.

Fruits should be eaten as a fruit meal, unmixed with other foods except lettuce and/or celery. Melons should be eaten alone.

Mineral Chart

ITS NAME	ITS FUNCTION	FOOD SOURCES
Calcium	Helps build healthy bones and teeth, aids blood clotting, maintains healthy nervous system	Green leafy vegetables, legumes, organic dairy products, molasses, nuts (particularly almonds), salmon, sardines, yogurt
Chromium	Helps maintain blood sugar level, aids metabolism of sugars for energy	Black pepper, cheeses, clams, corn oil, meat, mushrooms
Copper	Helps build healthy bones and teeth, aids healing processes, aids mental processes and emotional health, helps build healthy blood	Avocados, cauliflower, legumes, molasses, nuts, raisins, fish, whole grains
Iron	Aids in production of red blood cells, helps with stress and disease resistance, necessary for proper growth in children	Blackstrap molasses, dark green leafy vegetables, eggs, fish, legumes, poultry, wheat germ, whole grains, alfalfa
Magnesium	Helps maintain proper levels of blood sugar for energy, aids in metabolism	Bran, brown rice, green vegetables, honey, kelp, nuts, spinach, alfalfa
Manganese	Necessary for enzyme activation, aids sex hormone production, aids fat and carbo-hydrate metabolism	Bananas, bran, buckwheat, celery, grains, egg yolks, legumes, nuts, pineapple, seeds
Phosphorus	Helps build healthy bones and teeth, aids cell growth and repair, helps energy production, aids kidney function, aids vitamin utilization	Eggs, fish, grains, meat poultry, yellow cheese, alfalfa
Potassium	Helps regulate healthy heartbeat, aids muscle use, helps as nerve tranquilizer	Apricots, peaches, kelp, seeds, figs, blackstrap molasses, beans, cabbage family, dates, raisins, fish, spinach, tomatoes, tofu, bananas, alfalfa
Selenium	Antioxidant, aids pancreas function, helps eyesight, aids tissue elasticity, builds sex hormones	Cabbage family, eggs, tomatoes, wheat germ, whole grains, onion, fish
Sodium	Aids nervous system, helps maintain healthy fluid levels in the body, aids muscle functions	Sea salt, organic milk, cheese, fish, alfalfa, celery
Zinc	Helps with burn and wound healing, aids carbohydrate digestion, necessary for health of prostate and other reproductive organs, aids metabolism	Fish, meat, mushrooms, onions, soybeans, spinach, sunflower seeds, wheat germ, whole grains (preferably sprouted)

Appendix

MORE RESOURCES:

The Cook's Thesaurus: http://www.foodsubs.com
- For those who love cooking, but occasionally need an ingredient for your favorite recipe that you don't have on hand.

Encyclopedia of Spices: http://www.theepicentre.com

Buy Organic - hemp items, all natural health products, children's needs, organic wine, bontanicals, wheat free, gluten free, vegan foods.
Check out: http://ecopromoscious.com

Paleo Foods Resource:
http://paleofood.com/Grass Fed Meat
http://www.grasslandbeef.com
http://www.grazinangusacres.com - New York State
http://www.polyfacefarms.com - Virginia
http://www.organicprairie.coop
http://www.organicprairie.com/
http://www.wholesomeharvest.com
http://www.blackwing.com/ - Illinois
http://www.alderspring.com/ - Idaho
http://www.grassfedtraditions.com
http://www.grassorganic.com - Tennessee
http://www.cowboyfreerangemeat.com/ - Wyoming
http://keuneorganicmeats.com - Wisconsin
http://www.foxfirefarms.com - Colorado
http://www.lgbeef.com/ - Colorado
http://www.meadow-view-farm.com/ - Vermont
http://www.steakburger.com - Texas
http://www.lacensebeef.com/ - Montana
http://www.bighornmeats.com/ - Pennsylvania
http://www.morrisgrassfed.com/ - California
http://www.tallgrassbeef.com - Kansas
http://www.americangrassfedbeef.com/ - Missouri
http://www.hearthealthynaturalbeef.com - Michigan
http://wallacefarms.com - Iowa
http://peacefulpastures.com - Tennessee
http://www.texasgrassfedbeef.com - Texas
http://www.herondalefarm.com/ NY
http://www.lobels.com/ - NY
http://www.goodearthfarms.com/ - WI
http://www.wagonwheelranch.org/index.htm - MD
http://www.sevensons.net/ - Illinois
http://backcountrybeef.com/ - CO
http://sojournersheep.com/ - Mass
http://ourfarmtoyou.com/ - MN

These links are subject to change - if you discover one that does not work, please let us know and by emailing us at:
info@handbooktohealth.com

To further educate yourself read:

- *5 Easy Steps to the Care and Feeding of Your Human Being.* Vivian Rice and Edie Wogaman. Colorado Springs, Colorado: Wild Rice Nutrition, 1999.

- *Healthy Urban Kitchen Cook Book.* Antonio Valladares & Jaime Larose. "A Simple, Step by Step System for Shopping, Cooking & Eating Healthy Foods"

- *10 Talents Cook Book.* Frank J. and Rosalie Hurd. Collegedale, TN. The College Press, 1968, 1985.

- *Empty Harvest: Understanding the Link Between Our Food, Our Immunity, and Our Planet.* Dr. Bernard Jensen and Mark Anderson. Garden City Park, New York: Avery Publishing Group, Inc., 1990.

- *American Vegetarian Cookbook* from Fit for Life Kitchen. Marilyn Diamond. Warner Books, 1990.

- *Spontaneous Healing.* Andrew Weil, M.D. New York: Fawcett Columbine, The Ballantine Publishing Group, 1995.

- *The Whole Soy Cookbook.* Patricia Greenberg with Helen Hartung. New Three Rivers Press, 1998.

- *The Uncook Book.* Elizabeth and Dr. Elton Baker. Saguache, CO Communication Creativity, 1980.

- *The Book of Tofu.* William Shurtleff and Akiko Aoyagi. Brookline, MA. Autumn Press, Inc., 1975.

Recipe Index

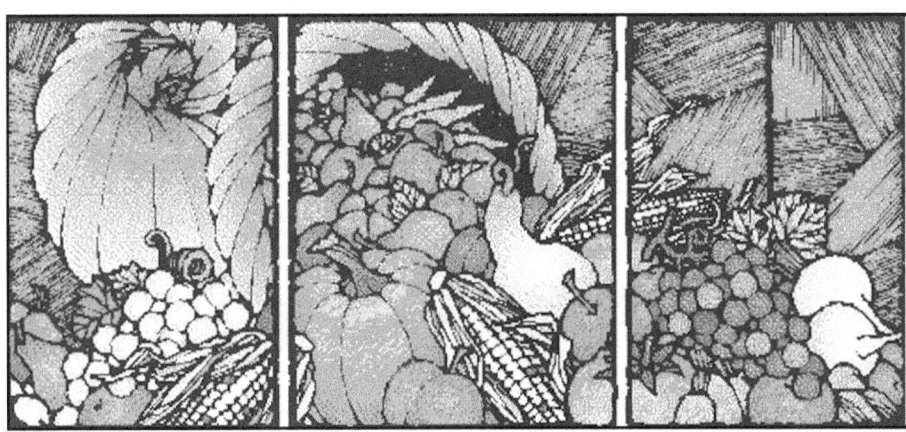

SOUPS

SALADS

VEGETABLES

MAIN DISHES

Carnivore ————————————*98*

Fowl, Poultry & Meat

NOTES

NOTES